# AGING BACKWARDS:
## *FAST TRACK*

ALSO BY MIRANDA ESMONDE-WHITE

*Aging Backwards*

*Forever Painless*

# AGING BACKWARDS: *FAST TRACK*

## 6 WAYS IN 30 DAYS TO LOOK AND FEEL YOUNGER

# MIRANDA ESMONDE-WHITE

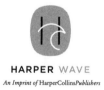

HARPER WAVE

*An Imprint of HarperCollinsPublishers*

This book contains advice and information relating to health care. It should be used to supplement rather than replace the advice of your doctor or another trained health professional. If you know or suspect you have a health problem, it is recommended that you seek your physician's advice before embarking on any medical program or treatment. All efforts have been made to assure the accuracy of the information contained in this book as of the date of publication. This publisher and the author disclaim liability for any medical outcomes that may occur as a result of applying the methods suggested in this book.

HarperCollins books may be purchased for educational, business, or sales promotional use. For information, please email the Special Markets Department at SPsales@harpercollins.com.

FIRST EDITION

Designed by Lucy Albanese

Library of Congress Cataloging-in-Publication Data has been applied for.

ISBN 978-0-06-285941-9

19 20 21 22 23  DIX/LSC  10 9 8 7 6 5 4 3 2 1

THIS BOOK IS DEDICATED WITH LOVE TO YOU ALL,
OUT OF MY DESIRE TO MAKE THE WORLD A
HEALTHIER, FITTER PLACE TO LIVE.

# CONTENTS

# PART II: THE MIRACLE OF MOVEMENT: THE 30-DAY FAST TRACK WORKOUTS

# AGING IS NOT INEVITABLE

As a child, I listened to the adults around me joke about getting old. I'd hear my young parents laughing about the fact that someday they'd need nurses and wheelchairs and endless medication. For my parents' generation, loss of mobility, poor balance, chronic pain, hip, knee, and joint issues, and low energy were inevitable. They simply developed a cheerful acceptance: *que será, será*—whatever will be, will be.

They lived very active lives, skiing, swimming, and gardening. But even all of those athletic pursuits wouldn't be enough to halt and turn back the aging clock. They didn't yet know (nobody yet knew!) that the weakness, immobility, and lethargy associated with aging are not normal; what *is* normal is to remain vibrant, active, and pain free well into our senior years. They didn't know that a few simple actions could help them remain pain free and youthful.

Back then, no one understood that if you didn't use muscles, they'd atrophy, your tissues would start to congeal, and movement would become stiff and painful. And unquestionably it would have been taboo to suggest that doing the wrong kinds of exercise would rapidly age the body.

Now we know differently! With the benefit of several decades of research, we know that inactivity—or the wrong kind of activity—is exactly what ages us fastest. And we know that we can turn back the clock just by learning how to move all of the muscles, connective tissue, and joints in our body.

When I was younger, I embraced my parents' attitude about aging. I assumed that I'd age in just the same negative ways as the generations who had gone before me. Well, something unexpected happened instead.

I didn't get older; I got younger.

I didn't get weaker; I got stronger.

I didn't develop more pain; I became pain free.

After suffering from broken bones, cancer, and all kinds of other medical issues, I'm now approaching seventy and I'm healthier and fitter than ever.

Much to my excitement, I recently literally *ran* up the 120-step Coba pyramid in Mexico and then I *skipped* down, not needing to hold on to the rope railing for aid. Despite their youth (all of my staff is under forty), some of the youngest members of my team struggled to navigate the steep, scary steps.

How is this possible?

I've spent years researching aging, and I know that aging happens only when we *let* it happen. When you move the right way, you have the ability to age backwards—to reverse stiffness and "stuck" tissue; get the juices flowing in your body; build strength, agility, and vitality—and stay young and limber for a very long time.

Now I also know how to jump-start the results more quickly than ever before.

## THE FAST TRACK

My love of movement inspired the start of my career at age ten. That's when I joined a professional ballet school. Later, I became a full member of the company of the National Ballet of Canada. After breaking my foot in seven places, at age twenty-one, I retired from the stage and opened a dance and fitness center.

For a long time, I was on the hunt for the perfect fitness program for my clients:

something that would help them build long, lean, ballet-dancer-shaped muscles; that wasn't as high impact as aerobics but equally strengthening; that could be done to classical, international, and modern music; and that was safe. I noticed too many of my clients experiencing injury and pain from the then-current high-intensity workout trends. When I couldn't find a suitable program, I decided to create one myself. (Yoga and Pilates weren't widely available yet.) The Essentrics fitness program is the result of many years of experimentation, scientific research, and fine-tuning. Designed to be done daily, by anyone, from cradle to grave, Essentrics is a simultaneous stretching and strengthening program to rebalance the full body in just 30 minutes a day. It is the basis for the popular television program *Classical Stretch,* which first aired on PBS in 1999 and continues to reach millions of Americans daily.

Since then, I've spent many years teaching, researching, and tweaking the fitness technique. I've worked with thousands of clients all over the world and have seen the dramatic and permanent changes in strength, weight, and body shape that people experience when they use Essentrics. Perhaps at no time are the improvements in appearance, health, and fitness more apparent than at my retreats.

Participants in my retreats range from age thirty to eighty. Many have lost hope for a healthy life due to years of rapid aging and chronic pain. At the start of a retreat, some participants show up in a state of depression, having silently given up on a better future. "This is normal aging," their doctors have said while prescribing joint replacement surgery or medication.

Over the course of seven days, including twice-daily exercise classes of 30 minutes each, I've watched as participants literally grow younger before my eyes. The changes are immediate: their skin starts to glow, the tension of chronic pain lifts from their brows, light shines in their eyes, their backs straighten, and their limbs move more fluidly. They feel real hope, many for the first time in years. Anne Legasse, age fifty-five, arrived thinking she might not be alive in ten years because of her health problems. Now she says she "can see my older self living to be a hundred like my grandfather did because I'm getting stronger every day." Le Rowell told me the retreats have been "a gift for aging well." At eighty-three, she is "standing tall, reaching those top shelves, and getting up and down with ease."

Watching these participants, I thought it didn't seem fair that only attendees learned how to permanently turn their lives around in such an accelerated way. I wanted to bring what made the retreats so effective to the widest possible audience and give everyone the same chance for a younger life. To do so, I knew I needed to create a program that:

- provides a simple starting point, a clear schedule, and a foolproof path.
- explains the breakthrough science behind the results.
- incorporates the most up-to-date science-based tools and strategies to make the program even more effective and the results stick, including the latest research on the power of slowness and visualization.
- allows you to see and feel improvement and track your progress.
- offers clear, achievable goals that encourage you not to miss a day.
- includes novelty to keep your interest and motivation high.
- transforms your total body and turns your aging process around immediately, no matter what specific condition or issue you may currently be living with.
- is designed to help you develop a daily habit of regular exercise.

Providing a clear structure, step-by-step guidance, and a 30-day incentive, the Fast Track plan is unlike any other program I've created. What you hold in your hands combines all of the elements present during the hundreds of retreats I've conducted, the thousands of classes I've taught, and the intense research I've done to integrate knowledge and movement into an easy-to-follow formula that will help you reverse unpleasant signs of aging such as stiffness, chronic pain, arthritis, and exhaustion while setting you on a path to feeling youthful for the rest of your life. Almost immediately, you'll start to enjoy real results:

- Improved posture
- Better balance
- Loose, supple joints
- Relief from chronic pain in your knees, hips, back, feet, shoulders, and hands
- Increased flexibility
- Renewed energy

You may be thinking, Miranda, if the participants in your retreats start to experience profound results in just 7 days, why is the Fast Track program for 30 days? Well, I've noticed that for some people, the sudden and significant changes they experience are enough to motivate them to continue exercising daily and keep growing younger and healthier. Others would return home, and despite the very best of intentions, would slowly slack off until they stopped exercising altogether. Watching this happen and hearing from other clients struggling to keep up a daily practice, I wanted to create a program that would motivate people to continue for years, never stopping.

There's been a lot of research on how long it takes to form a new habit and studies have shown it can take anywhere from 21 days to more than 2 months for a new behavior to become effortless and second-nature—something you fall into as naturally as brushing your teeth. Working with my clients, I've found that 30 days is just the right amount of time to set you up for a lifelong habit of daily exercise and give you the kind of life-changing results to make you look forward to it. And it's only 30 days—a month! Like a lot of people, I'm very goal oriented. Hopefully you are, too. The Fast Track program is designed to make great progress in a month—and it works. Give the program those 30 days. I know you can do it and you'll be glad that you did.

### Fast Track Is For You

Nothing has been more fulfilling in my life than watching and hearing about people whose lives have been turned around through regular correct movement. The Fast Track plan is for *everyone*—young or old, athletic or sedentary. It is for complete newcomers and for those who are already familiar with my work. Perhaps you've taken an Essentrics class, seen my PBS specials, or read one of my books. I've designed the Fast Track plan to offer you tremendous new benefits as well.

### Newcomers

Welcome! The Fast Track is the perfect place for you to start aging backwards. Don't worry about the exercise! When you're doing the right exercises correctly, exercise will feel good, both while you're doing it and afterward. Newcomers often tell me that they started feeling good the moment they start the exercises. Even people who said they hated exercising told me that their bodies seemed to be saying, "More, more, more!"

What surprises people most is that often they don't feel any muscle soreness after exercise, and if they do, it is mild. This tends to be very different from their previous experiences. Soreness is not a sign that you've done a great workout! Actually, soreness is a sign that your body is being forced to do something beyond its level of strength or flexibility. If you give your body a chance to develop strength and flexibility by working at your level, you will advance much faster.

Another cause of regular soreness after exercising is that few workouts are designed to rebalance the full body. The Fast Track workouts, on the other hand, are designed to fully rebalance the body and to prevent pain. Rebalancing the body is one of the basic principles of these workouts. Essentrics is about never, ever being in pain; it's about respecting and honoring your body and listening to its very important message of pain. Be patient and don't push your body into an injury. Let's discard the tired old maxim "No pain, no gain" and substitute a new one: "No pain!"

The Fast Track plan aims to find the perfect balance of enough, but not too much, exercise. If you wish to have a strong, mobile, pain-free body, then the path to achieving that goal is through moderation, not extremes. Exercising in moderation requires intelligence, knowledge, and discipline. In this book, you will learn why your body reacts badly to the extremes of either too much or too little exercise. Contrary to our usual view that moderation is mediocre, moderation in exercise is actually the only path to a pain-free active long life. Overexercising often leads to chronic pain, injury, and rapid aging, as does underexercising. Moderation will keep you youthful and vibrant no matter what your age.

Thanks to moderation, I feel younger, more energetic, and fitter at sixty-nine than I did in my twenties and thirties when I was a professional ballerina and aerobics instructor.

## Friends

I hope you've already experienced the amazing benefits of Essentrics. Perhaps you've tried some of my age-reversing workouts from my first book, *Aging Backwards*, or my pain-relieving workouts in *Forever Painless*. Over the years, readers and clients have shared their incredible successes with me, as well as their challenges. One of the biggest is maintaining motivation. The Fast Track plan is my reply: a turnkey program that offers accelerated benefits, total body transformation, and my most time-tested strategies to keep you motivated.

In Fast Track, you'll find:

- A kick-start to get you back into a regular exercise routine. If you've taken a break from daily movement, for whatever reason, Fast Track will get you back on track—and help you stay there.

- Ways to push through an Essentrics plateau. Are you regularly doing an Essentrics workout but don't feel you're seeing improvement? (Though you may not feel it, if you are doing the movements correctly, you are!) Use the Fast Track to refresh your routine and the large, complex movements to recharge your body and brain.

- New total body workouts. These workouts are completely new and they are not condition specific. No matter what your health goals or if you have an achy shoulder, stooped posture, or lower back pain, these workouts provide a complete reboot. Your whole body will feel better. I know that many folks turn to my workouts to ease a particular ache or pain, and when it's gone, they stop doing the exercises. If this is you, please know that Essentrics is of benefit to you always, every day, even if you're feeling good and pain free. Try these workouts and experience how much better you can still feel.

- New tools to amplify the power of these and all of my other workouts so you see results faster. These include the questionnaire I use with my clients to help you remember your body's history, discover the root causes of the pain or discomfort you've been feeling, and enable you to "go back in time" and finally heal. There are also visualization prompts with each exercise to help you perform them better and boost your brain health.

- Methods to maintain your motivation, for these 30 days and beyond. I know it can be a challenge. I've included my most effective strategies to keep you inspired. The results are the best motivation!

This book can be used as a reference for many years to come. I hope you turn to it again and again, both to explain changes that may be happening to your body and as an exhilarating guide to the life-changing potential of the Essentrics approach.

## LET'S GET MOVING

In the first section of the book, "Grow Younger Now: The Six Ways to Fast Track Aging Backwards," I'll share the program's secret sauce. It has taken me decades of research and working with scientists and students to identify the ways to make age reversal smarter, faster, and more effective. Understanding why these six ways are essential and how they work serves two purposes: motivating you to do the exercises each day and making the program more powerful.

Experience has shown me that the only way to motivate a person to commit to regular exercises is to give him or her a reward. I'd like you to consider the solid scientific proof supporting each of these ways your reward. I've witnessed the light in the eyes of my retreat participants as they grasp the science behind what was causing their aging, their pain, their arthritis, and their sedentary habits. Knowledge is a powerful motivator. Once you understand how your body works, why correct exercise is the only permanent way to reverse aging, and how you can easily and effortlessly make it a part of your daily life, you will become excited and motivated to exercise. You'll feel confident knowing that the exercise will pay off and reverse the signs of aging. With that assurance, you'll look forward to doing 20 to 30 minutes a day of exercises.

In addition to explaining the science behind the six ways, I explain how to use the science while doing the exercises to improve your results. Science remains theoretical until it is brought to life, in this case through movement. I'll show you how to put the theory into practice.

All of the six ways must be in place for the program to work. They are designed to work together, and so half measures or modifications don't work. If you don't follow all six of the ways, you will not age backwards at all but very likely age forwards. I've designed the program to make this effortless and easy for you. Just follow the program as written, paying particular attention to the instructions in the workouts, and you'll be incorporating all six ways to reverse the common signs of aging and become more vibrant, active, and pain free.

I have packed this plan with as many tools as possible to help you succeed, and the questionnaire in chapter 8, "Know Your Body: What's Your Aging Story?" is one of the most powerful. It's always surprising to me how often people misremember their medical history. It's common to disassociate your past health issues from your present aging process. The questionnaire will help you to acknowledge old pains and injuries so that you can progress forward to a new vibrant life. You have to fix what is wrong, if it is still causing a problem, in order for you to be free to move forward. If you don't know the original cause of your discomfort, it is much harder to fix it. This questionnaire will help. Please don't skip it.

Chapter 9, "Before You Begin: Set Yourself Up for Success," will tell you everything you need to do to prepare for the workouts.

Now to the workouts. There are two different levels:

1. The Fast Track 30-Day Starter Workout for what I call beginner-beginners, in chapter 10. This workout is for people who self-describe as being in poor physical condition or are recovering from an injury. If you've been struggling with chronic pain, haven't exercised for some time, or consider yourself to be in really poor shape, the Starter Workout is the smart place to begin. Try this level for 30 days and stay on it as long as you're comfortable. Some folks stay here for a long time, until they're ready to try the Core Workouts.

2. The 30-Day Fast Track Core Workouts for active adults in chapter 11 are for everyone else. If you are reasonably active, these workouts will be appropriate for you.

If you are unsure of your level of fitness, try the Starter Workout first, and if you find it too easy, go directly to the Core Workouts in chapter 11.

The Starter Workout is aimed primarily at the lubrication and release of congealed fascia, immobile ligaments, and tight muscles. It's a workout that is very easy on the body, so much so you might even wonder if anything is actually changing. The answer is yes, yes, yes. Your muscles and fascia will be gently hydrated with no possibility of any injury. The *inside* of your body is changing radically, and that's what counts.

The Core Workouts are comprised of three 10-day workouts. Each workout is divided into two parts. The first part consists of standing and chair exercises for full-body stretching and strengthening (30 minutes) and the second part is floor exercises for toning (15 minutes). The first part of stretching and strengthening is compulsory. The second part, for toning, is optional. *Never skip the first part of each workout.*

The Core Workouts are full-body workouts designed to safely unlock your body, step by step. The 10-day workouts proceed progressively, each building on the gains of the one before it.

Don't be deceived by the simplicity and seeming ease of these workouts. They may seem easy to do, but at the end of a month, you will find yourself with a spring in your step, feeling more energetic and stronger than you have in years. The deliberate, careful tempo we emphasize lubricates fascia, increases flexibility, and loosens blocked scar tissue that interferes with your ability to move through the natural muscle chains of your body. Once the natural muscle chains are liberated, strengthening muscles becomes much easier. You will be amazed at how rapidly your energy, strength, and vitality improve.

I've also provided 8 mini-workouts that I recommend you sprinkle like little jewels throughout your day. Not only will they boost your Fast Track results and generally keep your body limber and supple, they'll get you into the habit of viewing everyday life as an opportunity to move. Remember, movement is the signature of youth, so move, move, and move some more! I do these mini-workouts constantly throughout my day, wiggling my hands, fingers, toes, and shoulders. The more I move, the better I feel. The more I sit, like I am doing right now as I type, the stiffer and more uncomfortable I feel in my hips, shoulders, and back. So I do these mini-workouts and instantly feel much better.

When I was creating the Fast Track program I wanted to be sure to include ways for you to "see" and mark your progress in a meaningful way. It's so motivating and empowering to record, in black and white, how far you've come. The assessments in chapter 13, "Mark the Change: Celebrate Your Progress on Day 1, Day 15, and Day 30," will make you feel as though you have your own personal trainer watching over you and celebrating your progress with you.

## TIME TO CHANGE YOUR LIFE FOREVER

The Fast Track plan offers a new way of living, a new way of understanding, and a new way of perceiving the full potential of our physical bodies. I am so grateful to have been able to share what I have learned with you. I know that if you follow the 30-day program, your life will change forever. Mine did!

*Miranda*

# PART I

# GROW YOUNGER NOW

## THE 6 WAYS TO FAST TRACK AGING BACKWARDS

How can we turn back the clock on aging so quickly and powerfully, reversing stiffness and pain and increasing mobility, flexibility, energy, and vitality? These six essentials or ways hold the key. By incorporating these components, the Fast Track program provides concentrated, effective, and full-body results in a very short time. It's helped me to become pain free and fit for decades, and I know it can do the same for you, no matter how old you are.

Understanding the fundamentals of the program will help you to get even more out of the workouts. Science has shown us that understanding *why* an action benefits us increases the effectiveness of the action. So in the chapters that follow, we will explore the mechanics of the program, which will not only enable you to better understand how the Fast Track plan can turn back the clock at the cellular level but also help you improve your body awareness so that you can perform the workouts correctly.

Knowledge is the first step in putting the Fast Track program into action.

# CHAPTER 1

## WAY 1

# REBOOT YOUR MUSCLES, BONES, AND CONNECTIVE TISSUE

To fast track aging backwards, we must reboot our musculoskeletal system, a combination of the individual muscular, skeletal, and connective tissue systems of our body. Doing so is the first way for a very important reason: It's our muscles, bones, and connective tissue that make us feel and look old when they get out of shape.

The muscular system includes 650 voluntary muscles (muscles under your control); the skeletal system includes 360 joints and 210 bones; and the connective tissue system includes fascia, tendons, ligaments, cartilage, and more. When the musculoskeletal system is healthy, we move with total ease and we feel young and vibrant. In addition to making us feel terrific, a healthy musculoskeletal system protects and enhances the health of every other system in the body.

When the musculoskeletal system is unhealthy, our organs behave sluggishly and we gain weight; lose our shape; suffer chronic pain, osteoporosis, and arthritis; have less energy; and are chronically stiff. We feel old.

To turn back the clock we must keep the parts of the musculoskeletal system vibrant and healthy.

## MUSCLES

*Muscles are the guardians of our youth. We need our muscles for strength, movement, the burning of calories, energy, and the maintenance of our body's shape. Healthy muscles are designed to alternate between a state of tension and relaxation. When muscles are locked in a state of permanent tension due to atrophy, poor posture, overbuilding, or poor alignment, we refer to that as a state of permanent stress—or distress! Permanent tension reflects unbalanced muscles, which are the leading cause of chronic pain, damaged joints, and disease.*

If we don't move our muscles sufficiently on a daily basis, they will atrophy, shrink, and die. When muscles atrophy, we lose mitochondria, the valuable calorie-burning furnaces that give us energy and regulate our weight. As muscles weaken, we also lose our ability to move easily, making us *feel* old.

Muscles are created to be equally strong *and* flexible. Muscle cells are tubular shaped with a sliding mechanism, somewhat similar to an old-fashioned telescope that shortens and lengthens as you pull on the telescope's shaft. As muscles contract, they pull the joints closer together. This is fine as long as they are capable of releasing the contraction and shifting into an elongated or lengthened mode. The trouble begins when muscles lose their ability to release the shortened or contracted phase of the "sliding telescope," leading to joint compression, joint damage, arthritis, and eventually joint replacement procedures.

You will notice how painful your neck feels after you hold it in a forward bend while working on a computer. Holding any position requires the muscles to contract and remain contracted (even if the contraction involves the lengthening of muscles, as is true when you bend your neck forward for any length of time). This tension-pain will get worse if you don't do some kind of reverse movement, such as straightening your spine, stretching your arms above your head, and rotating them behind you. Being permanently locked in the shortened contracted phase of the "sliding telescope" is being permanently locked in a state of tension, or dis-ease . . . disease. Being in chronic tension is both unhealthy and uncomfortable.

There are a seemingly infinite number of ways to unbalance your muscles. Two of the most common ways muscles lose their ability to release the shortened position are because of disuse and strength training.

A sedentary lifestyle permanently shortens the muscles through atrophy and shrinkage. Muscles that are rarely stretched will permanently lose their ability to lengthen. The human body is efficient, and when we don't continue to perform a certain movement, over time the body will stop making those movements available to us. This is why sitting around too much causes you to lose muscle.

It's also why many people lose their flexibility as they build muscle in weight training or impact sports. Weight training and impact sports strengthen the muscle *by* shortening it. And while we know that strength training can protect our muscles and prevent falls as we age, the hidden secret in the fitness world is that many strength-training programs actually cause many of the injuries of aging like tendinitis; rotator cuff damage; and knee, shin, and ankle pain. These are all conditions of unbalanced action within the cylinder of the muscle cells.

In addition, the tight, shortened, bulky muscles developed in most strength-training regimes reshape the body. This bulky look comes with a price tag of compressed, tight, and damaged joints. Muscles cross over joints, so tight muscles translate into immobile joints! After a decade or so of compression, joint damage becomes arthritis, which may eventually lead to joint replacement.

Whatever the cause of permanently shortened muscles, the chronic pain is the same!

## The Fast Track Muscle Reboot

To be pain free and healthy, we must maintain our muscles' full range of motion. In order for us to age backwards and remain youthful no matter what our age, each of our trillions of individual cylindrical muscle cells needs to slide effortlessly from their most contracted to their most elongated length. The exercises of the Fast Track workouts are designed to do just that, transforming your muscles at the deepest cellular level. To achieve muscle cell transformation requires slow, deliberate movements. As you are doing the movements in these workouts, imagine releasing millions of strong, healthy muscle cells with each twist and stretch.

The Fast Track rebalancing, realigning daily exercises safely reboot all 650 of your muscles (it's easier than it sounds!) so aging never has to happen to them and they can stay strong and vibrant well into your senior years. These exercises:

**Prevent atrophy:** We need every muscle cell in our body to be healthy and moving. Only a full-body program like Fast Track will maintain the whole body and prevent muscle atrophy. Walking and machine training don't focus on maintaining or gaining the essential sliding action within the individual cell that is necessary to keep us young. Rather, they focus primarily on shortening the cell.

**Strengthen and stretch:** The Essentric exercises that comprise this program simultaneously strengthen and stretch the muscles in the same movements. To turn back the aging clock, we need our muscles strong *and* flexible. In the fitness field, there is a disproportionate focus on strength training as opposed to flexibility training. There is a long-held false belief that flexibility training is a waste of time because it won't prevent injuries, increase strength, or improve performance. This is only true if you are talking about passive stretching, as in massages or traditional hold-and-wait stretches. But this notion is dead wrong when it comes to Essentric exercises, which are done in constant motion. This is because any time you move your own body, strength is required because your body is a weight. Any time you lift any weight, some degree of strength is required. The method of flexibility we use in these Fast Track workouts adds incredible dynamic strength to the muscle while training the muscles to move comfortably through the full length of the "sliding telescope" between tension and relaxation.

And while we have 650 voluntary muscles—for example, the biceps, the quadriceps (quads), and the gluteus maximus (glutes)—we also have involuntary muscles (muscles over which you do not have control) such as our cardiac (heart), intestinal, and arterial muscles. As we strengthen our voluntary muscles, they automatically engage and strengthen the involuntary muscles (muscles over which you do not have conscious control). Any doctor will tell you that exercise is essential for keeping our cardiovascular system strong, but most leave out the fact that exercise is equally essential in keeping our digestive, intestinal, immune, and nervous systems healthy as well.

**Lengthen:** Fast Track workouts are eccentric exercises, strengthening the muscle by lengthening it. They reverse the compression on the joints, relieving joint pain, preventing and reversing arthritic pain and damage, and (possibly) preventing joint replacements.

# THE SCIENCE FICTION INSIDE

The activity inside of a muscle cell looks like science fiction. It's mind boggling to watch as a bulbous neuron synapse hovers over the surface of our muscle cells like a UFO, never actually touching the surface. Magnetic poles are reversed to open parallel portals in the neuron synapse hovering above the muscle. There is a chemical exchange of potassium and calcium between the neuron and the muscle through these portals. The chemical exchange triggers an entire cascade of chemical, neurological, and physiological reactions leading to a simple muscle contraction. This little futuristic performance is carried out millions of times daily as we conduct our lives.

## THE SKELETAL SYSTEM

*Our skeleton, which is made of 210 bones and 360 joints, is the scaffolding of the body, giving us our basic shape; tall, short, fine-boned, thick-boned, or stocky. Our bones may affect the way we look, but it's the strength of our bones that should concern us.*

Healthy bones are similar to healthy tree branches: they're very strong, yet they can give under pressure to prevent snaps or breaks. Unhealthy bones, similar to unhealthy branches, become dehydrated and brittle, breaking easily. Even the slightest pressure or awkward movement can cause brittle bones to snap, as can happen to people who suffer from advanced osteoporosis. It's also well known that the brittle bones of an elderly person are particularly vulnerable to breaks, which often happen should they fall.

To maintain or regain strength, hydration, and flexibility in all 210 bones, each and every one needs to be stressed or challenged. Stressing bones is relatively simple. Some experts recommend doing weight-training exercises: free weights or machines. I have two complaints with that suggestion. The first is that free weights and machines can stress only a limited number of our 210 bones, resulting in an imbalance. The second complaint is that the moment you pull or lift an exterior weight, the muscles of your shoulders contract, or shorten, compressing the shoulder joints. That's a physiological law and can lead to arthritis, rotator cuff injury, and other types of shoulder pain.

High-performance athletes do a lot of weight training, but most of them suffer from premature joint damage and need joint replacement surgery at young ages. Most high-performance athletes retire due to considerable pain in their late twenties and early thirties. The opioid epidemic has reached deep into the professional sports world, and damaged joints are the primary cause of these athletes' pain. I was a professional dancer, racked with pain from the age of ten until I retired, and so I understand the zaniness of an athlete's mentality. But I don't understand why any sane adult would choose to train like a professional athlete, especially after learning that the results of that kind of training are so devastating.

In addition to strengthening the bones, realigning the joints is essential to aging backwards. The alignment of our joints plays a major role in how well—or poorly—we age. Arthritic joint disease and the need for joint replacement are often caused by poorly aligned joints.

This emphasizes the need to focus on joint alignment in every exercise that we do. Joints are held in place by ligaments and moved by muscles. When the alignment is off, the ligaments around the joint are pulled off center and weaken. The muscles surrounding the joint reshape themselves, with some muscles working overtime to support the *off-center* joint while the others that are no longer being used weaken and atrophy. Connective tissue, such as the fascia, surrounding the joint also gets reshaped, creating an *off-center* fascia sleeve. The cartilage of the lopsided joint begins to wear down. All of this poor alignment leads to chronic pain and arthritis.

When the joint alignment isn't fixed, the ripple effect of damage to the surrounding muscles, fascia, and cartilage continues. The damage is accompanied by different degrees of joint pain, which often interferes with our daily routine and personal care. Dressing, bathing, cooking, driving, and working may become painful—or impossible. Poor alignment is so common that osteopaths and chiropractors spend their entire careers aligning joints.

To understand proper, or what I call "clean," joint alignment, you must know how muscles are situated in our joints. In order to bend and then straighten, joints are usually positioned in matching pairs. To bend our torso or the twenty-seven joints of our spine, we have two major matching pairs: the abdominal muscles at the front of the torso and the erector spinae group at the back of the torso. The erector spinae bend us backward while the abs bend us forward. Another obvious matching pair is the biceps and triceps, which cross over two joints, the elbows and shoulders. The biceps run along the top of the upper arm, and the triceps run along the underside of the arm. The biceps bend the elbow as they contract, while their matching pair, the triceps, relax and lengthen in order to permit the bend. They act like the up and down pulley belt of an escalator: The top part of the belt pulls the stairs up, while the bottom part pulls the escalator down.

In order to keep our joints well aligned, we must keep the muscles of the matching pairs well balanced, equally strong and flexible. If not, one of the muscle groups will overpower the other and pull the joint out of alignment. Imagine how dangerous an escalator would be if one side of the stair was higher than the other. Or if the bottom part of the escalator belt gets jammed, the upper part won't be able to move either. When we complain about having stiff joints, it's because the natural give-and-take *isn't happening.* An osteopath or chiropractor can put the joints back into alignment, but if our muscles are unbalanced, the moment we get off the treatment table, they will rapidly pull the joints back out of alignment.

# GOOD ALIGNMENT BEGINS WITH THE FEET

When someone calls attention to your posture, what's the first thing you do? Chances are you focus on straightening your spine. You'd actually be better off paying attention to the alignment of the 27 bones in your feet, and how the ripple effect of their poor alignment is spiraling up your legs and impacting your full skeletal alignment.

You can easily tell if the joints of your feet are out of alignment by checking the heels of your shoes. If there's a worn-down wedge shape on the heels, that means you have poor foot alignment. If the sole of your foot tilts away from your body, you have foot eversion. If the sole tilts toward your body, you have foot inversion. In order for you to be able to stand on the full soles of your feet, the matching pairs of your ankle and leg muscles must be equally as strong as they are flexible. If one muscle group is weaker than the other, it will pull your leg and foot inward or outward, leading to foot inversion or eversion.

Our feet are our foundation. If the foundation of a building is crooked, the whole house will be off-balance. Poor foot alignment will cause a ripple effect of poor skeletal alignment from your ankles through your knees, hips, and spine. Clean foot alignment is essential for good posture.

### The Fast Track Skeletal System Reboot

To maintain a healthy skeletal system, bones must be strong and joints well aligned. The Fast Track program is designed to do both. These exercises:

Strengthen: When clients first come to me, I ask, "Which muscles and bones don't you want to strengthen?" The answer is pathetically obvious; they want to strengthen them all!

Exactly.

The simplest and most effective way to recruit and stress all 210 bones is by doing large, full-body movements using the weight of your body as the load on the bones. Large movements that sweep from the floor to the ceiling while twisting and bending the full spine will effectively load and stress every bone in your body. These large sweeping movements also drive blood into the bones, delivering calcium and strengthening them. Making large movements is a powerful way to maintain and rebuild bones.

You will find these large, full-body exercises in all the Fast Track workouts. If you have limited mobility at first, don't worry. Over time, you will gradually gain strength and flexibility, making you capable of sweeping, twisting, and reaching farther. The larger the movements you make, the greater the bone-strengthening benefits.

Realign: Picture a loose door hinge. Something as small as a loose hinge can ruin the easy swinging action of the door, even leading to damage of the doorframe itself. The solution is as simple as screwing the hinge tightly to the frame. Like the hinge of the door, poor alignment in our body can be corrected by simply rebalancing all of our muscles and then training the muscles to support their joints in the correct place. Every workout in this book will rebalance and realign your muscles and joints.

Bear in mind that this takes time and feels awkward at first. The body is so used to our bad habits that correct alignment will actually feel wrong! And for sure correct alignment will throw you off-balance until you have strengthened and lengthened all the surrounding muscles. Poor alignment is reinforced by bad posture or poor walking habits, which take time to correct. On the encouraging side, remember that the human body is alive and designed to rapidly rebuild itself. Don't give up. With patience, you will see improvement and enjoy the many positive benefits clean alignment brings to you—more energy, less or no pain, and relief and healing of joint disease, to name a few.

Use a mirror to check your alignment while exercising. You'll be amazed how crooked your body is. Seeing it in a mirror will help you to catch your poor alignment and change it. It's normal if your body is incapable of aligning certain joints because of poor flexibility or a feeling that your joints are blocked. Don't worry. Keep trying, but don't force it. It could be caused by hardened connective tissue that will melt if you keep practicing.

It doesn't matter how long it takes to nudge your joints into correct alignment. What matters is that now you know to be aware of your alignment. And I hope it comforts and encourages you to know that through gentle regular exercising, poor alignment can be corrected.

## CONNECTIVE TISSUE

*Easy movement, no matter how small, depends on well-hydrated connective tissue. Fascia must be capable of slipping and sliding and ligaments must be capable of bending. To support the body and supply rebound energy, connective tissue must maintain its natural dynamic web by being strong and hydrated.*

Connective tissue is, by definition, tissue that connects every part of the body to every other part. This tissue comes in many forms: liquid, soft, and firm. For many years, Western anatomy textbooks posited that our bodies are held together with sheets of thick, dense connective tissue. Doctors viewed this tissue as inert packing material. Starting almost twenty years ago, Dr. Helene Langevin, working with her colleagues at the University of Vermont, began to prove that this connective tissue is in fact quite alive and very reactive to outside forces. Langevin and her colleagues showed that when you inserted acupuncture needles into specific areas, strands of the connective tissue would respond by wrapping around the needle. Then when the needles were removed, the connective tissue—in this case, fascia—would unwind and release substances like adenosine triphosphate (ATP), a compound that supplies energy to a cell, and immune system chemicals, sending signals that would radiate out beyond the local area to other areas of the body.

Langevin and her colleagues were fascinated by this work and kept going. If one type of mechanical manipulation (acupuncture) had this kind of impact on fascia, what would happen to fascia during another type (stretching)?[1] To study this, the scientists devised an ingenious method of teaching rats how to do yoga. They would pick the rats up by their tails, which would trigger an innate impulse for the rats to grab onto something with their front legs, such as the edge of a table or the bars in a cage. Doing so would automatically allow the animals to stretch out into an elongated state, similar to a human's yoga pose. Working gently and gradually, the researchers taught the rats how to increase their endurance, until eventually the rats were doing this "rat yoga" in a relaxed state for up to ten minutes at a time. This allowed the researchers to study the effects of "yoga" on the fascia—and what they found was truly amazing.

Once the rats were fully trained, the researchers induced a tiny amount of inflammation in the rats' backs. They found that the inflammation would resolve itself much faster in the rats that stretched than in the rats that did not. It turned out that the rats that stretched had more resolvins, a type of molecule that helps turn off an inflammatory response so that it does not become chronic. The connection was very clear: The externally applied biomechanics of stretching directly influenced the internal biochemistry of inflammation. (You'll be happy to know that the rats were eager to do their daily yoga just like people.)

What was even more exciting, when the researchers repeated the experiment with mice who had tiny tumors, they found that the mice who stretched had higher amounts of resolvins, which may help our bodies sweep away tumor cell debris. In addition, other researchers had already proven that tumors tend to adhere more easily and grow faster on stiff connective tissue—and tumors also excrete factors that increase the stiffness of the tissue. "The cancer increases the stiffness, the stiffness helps the cancer grow," says Dr. Langevin. Therefore, interrupting this positive feedback loop could help prevent cancer. By keeping the connective tissue limber with stretching, we might be able to stop cancer from getting started.

In the last twenty to thirty years, we have begun to understand more and more that mechanical forces interact with every single biochemical process of the body, from every single molecule within the cell, to cell division, to the functioning of organs, to the whole body. "At every single level, there's an interaction between the biochemistry and the biophysics," says Langevin. "We used to think that cells were these little bags that were just floating along. Now we can see that if we apply tiny force to the side of a cell, we can witness the molecules come apart and come back together, docking in and out of their receptors." This awareness points directly to the power of healing modalities such as massage, acupuncture, physiotherapy, and stretching, which tap into the power of biomechanics to influence biochemistry. These findings are reason for big hope: If we can keep our connective tissue limber, we may be able to prevent cancer from getting a foothold. If we can help tap into our body's innate resolvin supply, we may help reduce inflammation. And very recently, researchers have uncovered what may be the missing mechanical link between stretching, our immune system, and our biochemistry.[2]

Clearly our connective tissue is vitally important to our health, and the medical community is finally beginning to realize it. Connective tissue is now categorized as the third member of the musculoskeletal system, and scientists around the world are diligently studying it.

Through their research, we've learned that stiffness is more often caused by congealed fascia and dried-up ligaments than by tight muscles. It even turns out that it's our connective tissue congealing and hardening that make us feel and look old.

These findings are revolutionary, so it stands to reason they would compel a change in the fitness industry. Not only must we strengthen and stretch our muscles and toughen up our bones, but now we must equally include connective tissue in our fitness regimens!

### Fascia

*Fascia must be capable of doing a slipping and sliding action necessary to keep the liquid between the many layers of fascia from gluing them together. When the fascia layers congeal, we have trouble moving and we feel stiff and in pain.*

Under a microscope, fascia, cellophane-thin stretchy sheets of tissue with a watery-fibrous layer between each sheet, look like layers of a cake with icing between the layers. This collagen-rich, stretchy tissue forms an uninterrupted three-dimensional web within our entire body. Fascia is a subset of connective tissue that surrounds every muscle, nerve, vein, organ, bone—everything. (It has different names depending on what part of the body it is coating, but it is all the same tissue.) Think of it as a sleeve around a muscle or a bag around a cell. It has varying thicknesses and sizes and can be roughly divided into two types: superficial and deep. Fascia envelops everything from an individual microscopic muscle filament to a whole muscle group, a full limb, and even large body parts. One of the largest fascia configurations in the body is known as the "trousers" and is composed of a massive sheet of uninterrupted fascia that crosses over the knees and ends near the waist, giving the appearance of short leggings or trousers. This sheet is thicker around the knees, thinner as it continues up the legs and over the hips, and then thickens again near the waist. When this pair of trousers made of fascia is healthy, it acts like a girdle, giving us an attractive firm body shape.

Large sheets of fascia help support our muscles and bones and act as stabilizers to maintain our balance. Some sheets start under our feet, wrap around our torso, and finish in our hands. Others crisscross our torso, helping us maintain our shape as well as our balance. These fascia chains were of great interest to Dr. Langevin and her research teams.

Their work has helped to prove that these sheets, bags, and strings of fascia help muscles transmit their force and convert that force into movement known as dynamic tension. This fact alone underscores how critical it is to retain mobility and hydration in the fascia if we want to stay feeling vibrant throughout our life. When fascia becomes dehydrated from lack of movement, it congeals and makes us feel locked down and stiff. But worse still is that we lose the dynamic rebound tension that gives our movements vitality and ease.

The fibers of healthy fascia present themselves in a crimp pattern that has been proven to be stronger, ounce per ounce, than steel. Fascia fibers, unhealthy and weak due to lack of use of muscles, become disorganized and lose their crimp configuration. When fascia deforms into disorganized patterns, the fascia loses its strength and we feel weaker because we have lost the dynamic rebound action found in the crimp configuration of healthy fascia.

When this happens, fascia behaves like an elastic band that has lost its elasticity. Remember fascia surrounds our muscles; it can give us either a toned shape or a saggy shapeless shape. Our choice! As the fascia "bag" weakens, our muscles, which are wrapped in fascia, have nothing to hold them in their shape! This is one reason weak muscles are soft to the touch.

Congealed fascia is also a major cause of many health conditions such as back pain. Back pain sufferers commonly say they feel a pinching sensation that leads to spasm and excruciating pain. This pinching sensation is often caused by fascia that has hardened like a wad of fat, known as scar tissue, creating blockages in the natural movement chains in our body. After a while when we do try to move, any movement will pull against the wad, causing inflammation and irritation. When this condition is at its most extreme, you will need a myofascial specialist to dig into the fascia.

Between the many layers of fascia is a watery, oily fluid that lubricates the layers, permitting a sliding action to occur. The space between the fascia layers is called the interstitium—what I call the "oily bath." Under a magnifying glass, the interstitium looks like a spider web, but using a microscope, you can see it is made up of tens of thousands of interconnected, fluid-filled tubercles that are in a constant state of "shape-shifting" as they adjust to pressure caused by any movements that we make. The collagen of the interstitium forms a strong and flexible mesh that absorbs shock and responds to forces from inside (such as breathing and digestion) and outside (such as exercise and massage), helping keep this fluid circulating through the body.[3]

At a recent Grand Rounds lecture at Brigham and Women's Hospital, Dr. Langevin described the interstitium as a type of sponge. The connective tissue fibers make up the outer mesh-like structure, with little pockets inside that are ready to be filled with liquid.[4] And just as is true with a water-filled sponge, when we twist or stretch it, we encourage the fluid to release and flow out, creating a negative pressure that allows new fluid to flow in again. This action helps maintain the hydration and slipping and sliding action of the fascia. Without it, the oily liquid becomes sticky and slowly congeals the layers of fascia together.

## Tendons

*Tendons attach muscles to bones, making movement possible. Healthy tendons are well hydrated and pliable, while unhealthy tendons are brittle and prone to tearing.*

Tendons are identical in their physiological makeup to ligaments, but they have a totally different purpose in the body. Tendons attach muscles to bones, so their pliability is dependent on the flexibility of the attached muscle. Every time we move, we automatically engage our tendons. As long as the muscles are not extended beyond their natural stretch potential, the tendons are safe from being pulled beyond their capability. Most people rarely stretch their muscles too much except in a sudden sports or car accident.

We have a self-protective mechanism in our body in the form of reflexes. Reflexes are designed to prevent injury to tendons (and muscles)—and they actually succeed 99 percent of the time. When they don't work, it's usually because the stessful incident happened so quickly that the reflex didn't have time to kick in. When a muscle lengthens or shortens too much, too quickly, as in an accident, the reflexes can't react quickly enough to prevent the tendons from being sprained or torn.

## WHY WE NEED HYDRATION

It is easy to confuse a need for hydration with the feeling of muscle stiffness. Connective tissue becomes gluey when it is dehydrated. Dehydrated fascia stops slipping and sliding, making movements feel tight and stiff. This is when a glass of water will instantly hydrate the fascia and we feel loose again.

But the fascia sleeve surrounding every cell in our body requires regular hydration to keep it supple and functioning effortlessly. This includes the fascia surrounding our heart, veins, and arteries, which require constant hydration to prevent them from hardening, leading to heart disease. In fact, every part of our body requires constant hydration to prevent it from drying out and becoming brittle. And staying young means keeping our connective tissue slipping, sliding, and pliable. Water is the lubricant. We don't want to dry up. We want to keep our cells plump and healthy through hydration.

Drinking endless glasses of water isn't enough though. The key to hydrating your tendons, muscles, and organs is *to move*. We need to exercise and move so that our cells send the message that they need water. If we don't move the body, the cells have no need to ask for water and will slowly become dehydrated and shrivel up. And we especially need to *do some stretching movements to drive the liquid into your tissues*. Movement replicates the action of a sponge; with each movement, cells expel and then absorb water. Stretching draws that water into the tissues, hydrating them, enabling them to slip and slide against one another. Stiffness results from dehydrated tissues becoming gluey and incapable of slipping and sliding. When we don't move, water bypasses the cells and flushes right through the body—and we remain dehydrated and stiff.

Every time you move, you automatically lubricate your connective tissue. A little bit of full-body daily stretching will keep your connective tissue hydrated, helping to prevent tears, stiffness, and atrophy.

### Ligaments

*Ligaments must be sufficiently pliable to permit us to bend our fingers, knees, ankles, elbows, and spines while also remaining almost rigid in form, as they are the stabilizers of our joints. This means that their maximum range of motion can be only between 4 and 6 percent in order to support the structure of the joints while permitting them to bend. Weak ligaments cannot support or stabilize a joint, making the joints prone to injury and giving the body an appearance and feeling of limpness.*

Ligaments attach and hold everything in your body in their correct place. Your bones, liver, kidneys, heart, and other organs stay in their designated places because of ligaments. Ligaments also support and protect the integrity of the joint itself. You may have heard of the anterior cruciate ligament (ACL) and the medial collateral ligament (MCL) in the knee joint; they crisscross the joint's interior to give our knees the ability to slightly sway side to side—but not too much. Ligaments look like tough thick leather. They are extremely strong and difficult to cut but they can be overstretched, sprained, and torn.

Ligaments attach each one of our 360 joints to each other. Some joints have more ligaments than others, and some joints have complex patterns of cross-weaving ligaments, to suit the needs of each different joint. For instance, the ankle needs different stabilizing ligaments than our individual spinal vertebra. In addition to attaching bones to bones, ligaments attach our organs to their place in the body. What we have to care about is the need for all of these ligaments to be lubricated.

Dehydrated ligaments harden, causing stiffness in the massive web of connective tissue embedded throughout our entire body. We feel as if we are aging rapidly, and we are! Ligaments are made up of the same crimp formation as all healthy connective tissue. The massive accumulation of ligaments found in our joints has the ability to give every joint an incredible gift of dynamic rebound power. The healthy ligaments can literally act as a trampoline, giving us a bounce to our step as we run down the street and a feeling of weightlessness as we bound up the stairs. When these ligaments are well hydrated, they help make all of our movements feel light and easy. We can smoothly transition from sitting to standing, get in and out of a car, reach and bend to access cupboards, and twist to dress. Healthy strong ligaments make life easy. With healthy, well-hydrated pliable ligaments, we will never feel stiff and old.

It's important to note that ligaments have a maximum range of motion of 4 to 6 percent, which means a ligament's stretch potential is almost imperceptible. Muscles, on the other hand, have a 75 percent degree of flexibility. This means if we stretch our ligaments, we will damage the crimp and make ourselves weak. What we do need to do is make them sufficiently pliable so that we can bend them—our knees, spine, fingers, toes, and ankles. This underscores the danger of stretching a ligament in the traditional sense. Ligaments should be "manipulated" only into carefully achieving their designated *pliability* (versus flexibility, which we do with muscles). If a ligament is stretched beyond its very limited range of motion, the crimp-like formation is destroyed, making ligaments incapable of ever recoiling to their original supporting length. When this happens, the joint, which the ligament was intended to support, becomes permanently unstable. This results in joint damage, because the ligaments no longer support the joint. You'll find the most common joint wobbliness or weakness in ankles, shoulders, and knees after they've been twisted from a fall or injury.

But also many people unintentionally overstretch their ligaments due to ignorance. I get upset when I see athletes stretching their Achilles tendons by placing their toes on a edge of a stair and letting their heel hang downward. Despite the fact that it is actually going to weaken athletes, this dangerous stretch is highly recommended by coaches and therapists who don't realize that using the full weight of the body to stretch the tendon will overstretch it and create weakness in the ligament's crimp. Other common stretches that have the potential to overstretch ligaments are pulling your wrist with the opposite hand or stretching your neck by placing your hand on your head while leaning it to the side. We forget how powerful our arms actually are; using them to stretch our wrists or necks is asking for ligament damage.

Sedentary folks and active people who have not moved all of their joints (which is many athletes) lose pliability in their ligaments. One way we lose our pliability is by wearing shoes all of the time. Shoes are designed to protect our ankles and feet by partially immobilizing them. Many sports shoes lock the foot in a right angle, virtually immobilizing the ankle and toe joints. This leads to a loss of pliability in the ankle, eventually eliminating its ability to flex or bend. I've come across this all too often with hockey players, skaters, runners, and squash players.

## STAMINA, INJURIES, AND ATHLETES

Athletes who suffer from immobile ankles often also have poor stamina and chronic injuries. The first thing I do when training athletes is get them to take their shoes off and exercise the feet. Within minutes they start to regain the range of motion in their toes and ankles. Only when their toes and ankles can move will their injuries heal and their stamina return. The loss of stamina was from a lack of pumping action in their calf muscles; the rigid ankles blocked their ability to stretch and release the calf muscle.

The calf muscle is known as the second cardiac muscle due to its large size and its distance from the heart. The more we bend our ankles and knees (with flexible ligaments), the more the blood can be pumped upward. If athletes cannot bend their ankles, they cannot bend their knees, limiting the pumping action needed to circulate their blood efficiently. The better the circulation, the more oxygen is pumped into the muscles and the greater the energy. Bending the ankles and knees gives athletes the ability to pump their blood efficiently throughout their system, increasing their stamina almost instantly.

When it comes to injuries, tight ankles limit the movement in the natural muscle chains from the ankle to groin. We know that lack of movement leads to drying, atrophy, and shrinkage of the muscle cells along the immobile chain. Any sudden movement, like a deep lunge or a wide stride, can overstretch the muscles along the shrunken chain.

The way to improve stamina and prevent injury is to reintroduce mobility into the ankle. As the ankle bends, it permits the knee to bend. This is how flexibility is introduced into the dried-up, atrophied muscle chain. The amazing thing is that muscles respond extremely rapidly to stretching. The pulling is relieved by newfound flexibility of the muscles, which in turn leads to the chronic injuries disappearing.

### Scar Tissue

*Internal scar tissue, often due to immobility, surgery, or an accident, is one of the leading causes of chronic pain and difficulty in moving. Untreated internal scar tissue is a major cause of aging.*

The term *scar tissue* is often used to describe various forms of bonded cells that inhibit movement of a muscle, tendon, ligament, or joint. The most common causes of scar tissue are from a tear in the soft tissue from an injury or surgery. There is another type of scar tissue caused from tissue that builds up as a result of immobility. When you don't move regularly, the fascia in the unused part of your body congeal, fusing together and creating a wad known as scar tissue (sometimes quite a large wad). You can often find wads of scar tissue in the rounded back of someone with poor posture, or the upper backs of people who lift excessive weights.

Scar tissue is found externally as well as internally. When it forms in a muscle group, it cuts off one part of the muscle chain from another. Imagine a dam. On one side of the dam is a body of water, and on the other side is dry land. Scar tissue acts like a dam, cutting off one part of the muscle chain from the hydration it needs to stay healthy and prevent atrophy. Scarred muscles create a domino effect that leads to muscle imbalance, joint damage, and chronic pain.

### Fast Track Connective Tissue Reboot

Over the past two decades, the scientific community has produced a great deal of fascinating research on connective tissue, proving how integral it is to the health of the entire body. What most research points to is that full-body stretching is the most efficient way to age-reverse fascia, tendons, ligaments, and scar tissue. The exercises in the Fast Track plan:

**Reboot fascia:** Weakened, congealed fascia makes us feel and look stiff and old. It's most frequently caused by a sedentary lifestyle in which unexercised muscles are permitted to slowly atrophy, causing the surrounding fascia to become gluey and rigid. Sitting sets us on a slippery slope where the less we move, the more the fascia congeals. The large slow movements in these workouts focus on maintaining healthy fascia. Do the exercises with the awareness that you are actively trying to decongeal glued fascia.

**Reduce stiffness:** Stiffness is a sign of aging, yet stiffness is not caused by aging! Stiffness is caused by not moving enough. Our fascia is not destined to suddenly become stiff as the years go by. The only reason our fascia congeals and becomes stiff is that we chose not to move! Take heart! In the Fast Track workouts, you will twist, turn, stretch, wiggle, and rotate your fascia so you should never feel stiff again.

**Relieve back pain:** In addition to congealing fascia, chronic back pain is the most common consequence of a sedentary lifestyle. When we sit a great deal, the back and hip muscles inevitably weaken, becoming prone to spasm. A spasm can lock muscles and fascia in excruciating pain for days at a time. When fascia cannot move, you cannot move. The fastest way to break the cycle of chronic back pain is with regular full-body stretching.

**Rehydrate tendons:** Tendons are automatically engaged every time we stretch or strengthen a muscle. A full-body daily workout will automatically engage your tendons, keeping them hydrated and healthy. As long as we do a non-aggressive full-body workout, our tendons are automatically hydrated every time we stretch our muscles.

**Rebuild firm, mobile ligaments:** Without regular exercise, ligaments lose their pliability, becoming dehydrated, brittle, and easily torn. To prevent that from happening, they require regular *pliability* exercises, gentle movements aimed at lubricating and rehydrating our ligaments. You will find many of these in the workouts. It may take days, weeks, or even months to completely regain the full pliability of your fingers, toes, and ankles, but be patient. You don't want to stretch the ligaments, just move them enough to keep them well lubricated and safe. They need to be exercised like every other part of the body, but very intelligently and carefully. The slow, deliberate movements in these workouts are specifically designed to return mobility and pliability to your ligaments safely. As long as you follow the Fast Track program as presented, change will happen.

Reduce scar tissue: The binding effect of internal scar tissue can be largely reversed with daily stretching. In order to do that, we must stretch the full body and break down the higgledy–piggledy nature of scar tissue buildup. The full-body nature of these workouts pulls the muscles in multiple directions, helping to sluff away scar tissue buildup. Studies have shown us that the more we stretch scar tissue, through either exercise or massage, the more mobility will be returned to that area.

# CHAPTER 2

# WAY 2
# RECHARGE YOUR BRAIN

In order to age backwards, we must keep our brains fit and vibrant and focus on our brain's health. *Use it or lose it* applies to the brain as well as the brawn!

Many of us worry that our minds will become feeble as we age. We worry about becoming forgetful and slow to comprehend, or suffering from a loss of long-term memory. Worst of all, many of us feel helpless to prevent the common aging-brain conditions of dementia and Alzheimer's.

These are reasonable worries, as we have seen the brains of loved ones and friends deteriorate as they age. It is obvious that our brain is as susceptible to atrophy and cell loss as any other part of our body. However, new studies are being published that prove that our brain is equally capable of growing new cells and maintaining our cognitive health as we grow older.

One positive side of aging in this period instead of fifty years ago is that our overall life expectancy has increased. With advances in medicine, we've experienced a decline in premature deaths due to certain chronic diseases. So we are living longer—and that's certainly good news.

On the negative side of the ledger, deaths due to Alzheimer's disease have increased over the past decade by nearly 87 percent.[5] For people over the age of eighty-five, there is a fifty-fifty chance of developing Alzheimer's. And even if we don't develop Alzheimer's, the thought of losing our ability to remember important dates, precious memories, and ways to perform our everyday activities is still a big fear. As a culture, we've become a little fatalistic about our cognitive health. We've grown to believe that a certain amount of forgetfulness is an inevitable part of aging. But while some people are more prone to developing Alzheimer's due to the inheritance of unfortunate genes, according to recent research, the progression of most cognitive decline can be reduced, delayed, or even prevented just by making simple lifestyle changes—including correct exercise.

One of the most exciting scientific conclusions of recent years was the discovery that basic movement can help grow new brain cells—and that complex movement can increase the number of new brain cells even more. Just as we can reverse atrophy in our muscle cells and improve our strength and flexibility, so too can we improve our cognitive functioning.

Until the late 1990s, scientists believed that our brain was fully developed by our adolescence—and from then on, it was all downhill. We'd be losing neurons thereafter, every decade. In 1998, scientists made one of the biggest discoveries of the twentieth century: They found conclusive evidence that neurons continue dividing and regenerating—a process called neurogenesis—well past our adolescence! This discovery has opened up an entirely new field of research for neuroscientists looking to speed up the rate of neurogenesis, thereby potentially helping stall or even prevent Alzheimer's and other types of cognitive decline.

How does this later-in-life neurogenesis work? The brain is made of billions of neurons, with trillions of connections between these neurons. By increasing the amount of certain proteins, known as *factors,* in the brain we can improve the rate at which these connections develop and grow and enhance the connections in our brain so that we think faster.

Brain-derived neurotrophic factor (BDNF), also known as "Miracle-Gro for the brain," is one of the key proteins (or factors) involved in enhancing the function of neurons, increasing their growth, and improving their ability to make these connections. Studies have shown that certain types of exercise increase BDNF in the brain.

When scientists first did these studies, they assumed that this new neural growth would take place in areas of the brain that controlled motor skills, such as the cerebellum. Studies of mice running on treadmills found that the farther the mice ran, the higher the levels of BDNF—but the levels increased most dramatically in the hippocampus (the area of the brain involved in learning and memory). Increasing the number of brain cells in our hippocampus may not only improve our ability to learn but also speed up the rate at which we grasp new concepts and make new connections in our brain—all of which can reduce our later risk of cognitive decline.

Armed with this discovery, experts set out to find what type of exercise would be best for the brain. For example, it stands to reason that you would not want to choose an exercise program that would increase the body's level of the stress hormone cortisol, which has been shown to decrease brain size. Any kind of forced exercise—overtraining, being yelled at, pushing through pain—can create stress in the body, joints, and brain, impacting our cortisol levels, which would have negative implications for our cognitive functioning. A certain degree of stress hormone can be exciting and good for us. The adrenaline rush you get when you see the finish line is certainly motivating! But the cortisol triggered by uncontrollable stress can increase levels of anxiety and depression, can lead to digestive problems, can cause disrupted sleep, and can even depress our immune function, making us vulnerable to other physiological changes—including, ironically, a higher risk for Alzheimer's and other chronic diseases.

So which types of exercise do increase levels of BDNF in the brain and help us optimize our cognitive functioning? For a sheer increase in the amount of BDNF, the research initially suggested that aerobic exercise was the ticket. The impact on BDNF levels in mice who ran on treadmills was certainly easy to study, and indeed, cardiovascular exercise has been shown to have a dramatic effect on our levels of BDNF in the brain. But placing one foot in front of another does not exactly challenge the brain's complexity.

What if you could tap into exercise's potential to increase BDNF *while* doing something mentally challenging—would that boost the effect? In a series of studies conducted at the University of Illinois, researchers compared the brain changes in a group of rats that completed a complex motor-skill learning task to those that ran on a treadmill. The number of synapses per neuron in both the motor cortex and the cerebellum was greater in the rats that did the complex course compared to those that just ran on the treadmill. This increase in synapses lasted for at least four weeks after the training was done.[6]

Another experiment from the University of Illinois found that rats that were taught complex motor skills that involved balance experienced a 35 percent increase of BDNF in the cerebellum, compared to the running rats, who had none. Clearly there's something to be said for choosing a program that challenges our cardiovascular system *and* our brain, improving our balance, agility, and coordination skills—like Fast Track.[7]

## FAST TRACK BRAIN RECHARGE

There's simply no need to resign yourself to cognitive decline. Exercise plays a major role in maintaining and building neurons and synapses, and the right kind of exercise can do it faster and with better results. Using complex movements and visualization, the Fast Track plan will efficiently keep your brain young and vibrant, not only preserving your brain's status quo but helping you become even *smarter* as you grow older. These exercises:

Involve complex movements: Complex exercises that involve twisting, turning, bending, and reaching like these Essentric Fast Track workouts, tai chi, and dancing have been proven to be very powerful stimulants to growing new brain cells. When you ask your body to move in complex ways, your brain has to figure out how to make all of the various body parts move simultaneously in these new patterns. Every time we contract muscles, we initiate these contractions in the brain. Even the mere thought of moving our muscles stimulates activity in the brain. Every single muscle contraction and release comes from a message in the brain—the more complicated the movement, the greater the activity occurring in the brain.

The full-body exercises of the Fast Track plan pump blood through your entire body, creating new blood vessels that also help spawn neuron growth. Large complex full-body movements by definition challenge your brain to manage the distribution of the weight of all 650 muscles and 210 bones to prevent you from falling over as you move. Brain-stimulating workouts like these simultaneously grow new neurons while putting new neural pathways to work strengthening those connections.

Learning is a survival mechanism that we use to adapt to constantly changing environments. When we follow an exercise regimen that nudges our body out of its comfort zone, by shifting from position to position and targeting our muscles from different angles, we challenge our brain to adjust and adapt our body in every position. One of the most inspiring things about this ongoing brain research is how it proves that no matter what your age, through movement you can strengthen your neural pathways, increase the number of neurons in your brain, and enhance your ability to learn and adapt. Don't worry if at first you feel confused by the workouts. Take comfort in knowing that this confusion is actually good for brain development! Learning has been and always will be a humbling experience, but the reward is well worth it.

If the moves seem too complex, don't give up! You want to rejuvenate your brain, don't you? Trust me, your brain will find a way to obey your command. It might take time, but that investment of time is actively combating dementia.

**The neuron-building power of visualization:** Once you've mastered the basic moves of the Fast Track workouts, you can increase their benefit by using visualization during your movements. For instance, while doing a specific exercise, imagine that you are lifting a feather or a huge bag of rocks. Your brain then has to adjust the tension in your movements to match the imagined weight. Visualization causes your brain to search out tens of thousands of sleeping motor neurons to figure out the difference in muscle tension required for lifting feathers versus lifting rocks. Muscles that had just been contracted are then relaxed, all because of the image in your mind. Many people have trouble figuring out how to relax consciously, but your brain is the boss and will figure out a way to obey the new command.

When following the workouts in this book, carefully read the captions, which will offer suggested visualizations for each exercise. These visualization commands are designed to rebuild brain cells and neurological pathways—and age your brain backwards.

# CHAPTER 3

## WAY 3

# REBALANCE YOUR BODY

To age backwards, the physical body must be balanced. All parts of the body should be capable of moving in total ease. No one muscle group should be capable of overwhelming another muscle group. No one part should be weaker or less flexible than another part. In a fully balanced body, all of the parts should work in perfect harmony.

Every muscle—all 650, not just the major ones—should move easily and be as strong as they are flexible. The skeletal muscles are layered like clothing on our body. The largest muscles are closest to the surface, such as the gluteus maximus (or glutes, for our bum) and the quadriceps (or quads, for our thighs). The muscles closer to the body's interior are naturally smaller. The smallest muscles are often referred to as the stabilizers, as they hold joints in their proper position. The stabilizers are as essential to maintaining our balance and preventing joint damage as the large muscles are to moving our limbs through space. Neither is more important than the other.

When we focus on building strength in the large muscles, such as the glutes, biceps, quads, and pectorals, by doing weight training, squats, chin-ups, and push-ups, over time, the major muscles overwhelm the smaller micro muscles. When the micro muscles aren't engaged, they slowly shrink and atrophy from disuse. The stabilizing muscles are no longer strong enough to do the job of protecting the joints. This leads to joint damage.

But it also creates another unseen problem: a loss of energy! We have 650 muscles that are designed to work in harmony with one another to make all movement effortless. However, if we are only using our major muscles, we are literally engaging only half the potential power we are born with. As the major muscles do all the work of moving our body around, they naturally tire easily. This is the definition of an unbalanced body.

But in addition to all muscles being as strong and flexible as their neighbors, the individual muscle cells must also be fully balanced. What do I mean by a balanced muscle cell? A balanced muscle cell works according to its design. A muscle cell is designed to slide in and out of its cellular sheath as it contracts and stretches. As the muscles are being exercised, the muscle cells must always maintain their ability to slide fully in a contraction and an extension in order to be balanced. Having balanced muscles means that not only are your muscle groups equally strong and flexible but that your individual cells are well balanced within their individual cell pods.

The most powerful regulating mechanism for our musculoskeletal system is the message sent from a damaged area to our brain, telling us something is wrong somewhere in our body. In other words, pain is an important message. Then we have to make a conscious choice whether we want to stop damaging our body or to willfully continue causing harm.

When we sit at a computer, we put stress on the hands, shoulders, and neck. If we sit all day, this repetitive stress unbalances our muscles, bones, and connective tissue. When we sit for prolonged periods of time, the immobility within the muscle cells of our necks, shoulders, backs, and hips leads to discomfort and pain. As we sit barely moving, with our back and shoulders drooping forward, the connective tissue slowly congeals, forming what will eventually become a hunched back. Hip muscles weaken, and all of this is soon followed by chronic exhaustion. This is how our daily lives lead us to having an unbalanced body.

When I was a professional ballet dancer with the company of the National Ballet of

Canada, I had a lot of fun, but as is true with many retired professional ballet dancers, the years of intense movement left me with a broken body at a young age. Being in the dance and fitness field all my life, I've witnessed firsthand how most popular sports and fitness activities cause many preventable injuries. When I started studying the impact of these exercises on the musculoskeletal system, it became crystal clear: They caused a lack of balance within the cells.

Carpal tunnel syndrome, a stress-related repetitive motion injury of the wrist, is a common injury in the corporate, dance, fitness, and sports worlds. Shin splints, shoulder and back pain, hip and knee joint damage requiring replacements, and labrum tears of the hip or shoulder joints (tears to the ring of cartilage surrounding the joint socket) are all caused by repetitive motion unbalancing the body. Most sports and fitness programs cause imbalance. Fast Track workouts are designed to rebalance any and all muscular imbalances.

## FAST TRACK BODY REBALANCE

A balanced body is a powerful one, full of energy and pain free. It is something that anyone at any age can achieve with a science-backed rebalancing exercise program. I view the human body as one large unit rather than a collection of isolated "target areas." Keeping all of the parts of your body equally balanced, right down to your cells, is my top priority.

To rebalance the body, you need to bring it back to life by exercising the *whole* musculoskeletal system. These Fast Track workouts:

- Engage all 650 muscles in strengthening and stretching at the same time so that they are all as strong as they are flexible.
- Move the 360 joints in every direction that each joint is designed to move.
- Are not repetitive.
- Work the major muscle groups with the micro groups. We keep the actual exercises gentle enough to ensure that the micro groups as well as the major muscle groups are worked.
- Involve constant twisting, turning, bending, and reaching in various directions and planes.

Rebalancing your body takes time, as each of the many layers of tissue, from fascia to muscles, responds to movement differently. But it will happen. You won't develop rock-hard, immobile muscles in this program, but you will develop firm, strong, long, lean flexible muscles that offer you full strength and mobility. By simultaneously engaging your macro and micro muscles, you'll also have more energy.

## WEIGHT TRAINING IS FOR PROFESSIONALS. ARE YOU ONE?

Many athletes and fitness aficionados train with very specific objectives in mind—run faster, jump higher, get thinner, burn calories. They also focus on specific body parts, such as strengthening the biceps or toning the glutes. Unfortunately, achieving a well-balanced muscular body is usually not one of their goals. It's not surprising, really. Very few people understand the importance of balance and prioritize it the way I do.

It's a shame because an unbalanced body is why there are so many injuries in the sports and fitness worlds, as well as for those who practice "unfitness" programs.

If you are ever in a gym, take a look at anyone who does a lot of push-ups or weights. Weight trainers will very likely have a rounded upper back, with their shoulders pulling inward. This is an indication of an unbalanced body; it's obvious to the naked eye that some of their muscles are overpowering others. We are designed to have liberated shoulders and upper backs, but if the muscles of the chest (pectorals) have been repetitively strengthened, the muscles' cells will permanently shorten, leading to a rounded back.

I do not believe that free weights and strength-training machines are necessary for the average person's strengthening requirements. While high-performance athletes require this type of strength training to achieve their goals, most of them live in chronic pain all their lives. Twenty-year-old athletes have the body age of sixty-year-olds. Chronic pain is one of the signatures of aging. It is not compatible with the goal of living a long, healthy, youthful life—and certainly not a part of aging backwards.

We cannot be both healthy and damaged; these are two totally incompatible concepts. You can be one or the other, but not both at the same time. Thankfully, many sports champions and Olympic medalists I've trained have come to understand that the more balanced their bodies are, the fewer injuries they will suffer and the less pain they will endure, and the more medals they will win.

If you are a normal person and not a professional athlete, your actual body is a weight. Your arms are already a sufficient weight to lift when trying to strengthen the shoulders and spine. You don't need to add additional free weights to strengthen your muscles. Your head is a weight, as is your torso. Bending and straightening your torso as you do side bends is a weight-lifting feat sufficient to healthfully stress all the bones and muscles along your spine. A wide tai chi plié knee bend puts plenty of weight and stress on the hips, knees, thighs, shins, and ankles—definitely enough weight to strengthen these bones and muscles. You don't need more weight than your very own body offers. In other words, your own body offers you all the weight that you could possibly need to safely stress and strengthen your bones and muscles.

You don't need to add weight, and in fact, using weights causes compression damage to the joints. The moment you lift a weight, even if it's only three pounds, the muscles contract, pulling the two bones of the joint close together, leading to compression of the joint. However, when you do the identical movement of lifting your arms without weights, you can actually relax the joint muscles and actively pull the muscles into a lengthened position. Fast Track, a weight-free program, will liberate your joints while strengthening your muscles in a lengthened position. Use your body as your weight, not machines or free weights, and you will get a strong, pain-free body.

# CHAPTER 4

## WAY 4

# EXERCISE PAIN FREE

Any fitness regimen is by definition assumed to make you fit. It shouldn't deliberately cause you pain, as pain is a message that something is damaging your body. Pain is a message that you should stop hurting yourself! If an exercise causes you pain, there are two things you should do: Stop doing it and ask yourself why. Pain isn't a sign of improvement. It's exactly the opposite. It's a well-known fact that exercising in pain causes more inflammation and often serious injury. Pushing your body further when you are already in pain sets you up for long-term chronic pain. Just to be clear, I'm not talking about discomfort or a feeling of exhaustion while exercising, I'm talking about an ouch-inducing, knifelike pain that makes you wince.

Nothing ages us more than chronic pain. If you are one of the 76.2 million Americans—one in four—who is suffering from chronic pain, then you know exactly what I mean.[8] And if you are an exercise enthusiast who pushes through pain during a workout believing in the false mantra of "no pain, no gain," then you are setting yourself up to join those ranks.

Pain makes you walk and move in a restricted, self-protecting manner. It takes the carefree bounce out of your step and closes you down, keeping you in constant fear of making the pain worse. Pain contracts the muscles of the injured, inflamed area, such as your knees or shoulder, as well as supporting muscles throughout your body, including in your face. Pain makes you wince and frown, giving you a permanent expression of tension and discomfort. In other words, chronic pain ages you.

But when our pain is relieved, that contracted facial expression literally disappears. We stop wincing and frowning, so our face relaxes, instantly changing from looking old and worn-out to youthful and glowing. One client told me that friends thought she'd had a facelift because she looked so much younger after a week of pain-free exercising. This age-reversing benefit to your face is nothing compared to the relief of actually being pain free.

Pain is a message designed to get our attention and let us know there is potential or real damage to our body. When the damage is minor—caused by a scratch or insect bite, for example—the pain message will be minimal. Major damage, such as a broken bone or a bad burn, generates pain messages that are off the charts. The intensity of the messages is designed to force us to pay attention and fix what is wrong.

The pain message triggers the amygdala, the brain's fear center, to release stress hormones to help deal with the emergency. If we stay in that stressed state for too long, as happens with chronic pain, the pain pathways in the nervous system become extremely deep and hard to escape.

In some cases our nerve fibers continue to fire, sending pain signals through the nervous system up to the brain, long after the injury has healed. This is known as *phantom pain*. The pain is real, but the damage to the body is not. In addition, the body's pain receptors may become more sensitive to pain, creating more frequent pain signals and triggering the release of more pain-causing neurochemicals. Persistent chronic pain or pain from a lifetime of multiple accidents or surgeries creates an unending pain loop.

To tolerate chronic pain, for days, weeks, years, even decades, many people readjust their lives to avoid provoking more pain, keeping the body in permanent protection mode. We protect ourselves to avoid pain, but by not moving, we bring about a cascade of side effects from a sedentary protected life. These side effects include congealed connective tissue, muscle atrophy, musculoskeletal imbalance, and more pain. And we feel old! Healing cannot take place in protection mode—so we get stuck in a catch-22.

Chronic pain is as complex as each individual who has it. However, the human body is not designed to be in pain. The pain message is intended to be only a warning signal that something is wrong; consequently we are supposed to fix whatever is wrong, and then the message will automatically turn off. It's not designed to stay on permanently. It stays on only because we aren't fixing the problem. The primary purpose of pain is to alert us to stop damaging our body. We're designed to heed the message and make a change. But so often, that's not what we do.

We try to block out the pain signal with medication. When the medication blocks out the pain, we can continue doing whatever activity caused the damage in the first place—and the injury and pain only get worse. We are not smarter than nature. We ought to trust what our body is telling us and stop doing what is causing our pain, instead of drowning out the message.

I don't mean to minimize anyone's struggle with pain. If pain wasn't tough to endure and to deal with, it wouldn't be such an intractable problem in the world. We wouldn't have an epidemic of chronic pain, and we wouldn't be in the middle of a crisis of opioid addiction. As I write this book, I am working with some of the world's leading pain researchers, and I can tell you with great assurance that the pharmaceutical world still doesn't have a clue how to reverse chronic pain. So don't feel bad if you haven't found the solution yet; even with billions of dollars invested in research, neither have the scientists! From my many conversations with pain scientists, I've learned that many now believe they have been looking in the wrong place for the cure to chronic pain. No amount of pharmaceutical chemistry will solve a mechanical problem with the body.

The solution to mechanical pain is through correct mechanical treatments that work on the *mechanics* of the body, such as Essentrics exercises. The only way to heal damaged muscles, bones, and connective tissue is to move them in a way that gently heals them; that means exercising in a pain-free mode.

## FAST TRACK PAIN FREE

There is only one mode in which to exercise without fear of injuring or damaging your body, and that is in a pain-free mode.

As a society, we have embraced being tough on ourselves as a winning philosophy. We respect and idolize athletes who push themselves through a finish line with broken bones and twisted limbs. The more blood athletes spill and the more bruises they endure, the greater our respect for them. This makes embracing this new approach to fitness of being kind to yourself and avoiding pain a difficult one to adopt. So I invite you to think outside the traditional box and consider the basic logic and science behind this approach.

Exercising in a pain-free mode is the fastest way to eliminate chronic pain by letting the injury heal. The brain is designed to self-protect every cell in the body, so when we exercise or move in a pain mode, the brain springs into a form of self-protection lock-down where no healing can occur. (Movement is medicine, so when the body locks down, it blocks movement!) When you exercise in a pain-free zone, the self-protection reflexes don't kick in, thereby allowing healing miracles from movement to happen to your body.

If you are presently living with chronic pain, the Fast Track plan is designed specifically for you. Nothing heals and reverses chronic pain better than being pain free while exercising. Know this: By exercising in a pain-free mode you can fully heal and reverse your chronic pain.

Exercising in a pain-free mode is also one of the safest ways to build strength, flexibility, agility, and endurance. Aren't these qualities essential to turning back the clock?

Over these next 30 days, do all of the workouts in pain-free mode. Never slip into pushing yourself through the pain; never tolerate your pain; never "suck it up."

If you do feel pain at any point during your workout, gently readjust *how* you are exercising, and return immediately to the intensity level you were at before the pain kicked in. Sometimes you may experience a moment of pain when your movements are too large or too rough—for example, your arms are too high or your knees too bent. Return to the height of lifting or degree of knee bending where you felt no, or as close to zero, pain. Always return to a place in the sequence where you find you are pain free, and use that as your base point. Some people may feel as if they're wasting their time by hardly moving—but throw that thought out! This is a very deliberate technique that will change your life forever. Give it a chance. These exercises:

Are empowering: Pain is the leading cause of doctor visits. Yet sadly, more than half of the people surveyed by the American Pain Foundation feel they have little to no control over their pain.[9] The Fast Track plan gives you control with a program that is a scientifically based solution to end your chronic pain.

**Heal the root cause of pain:** In contrast to the fleeting relief of a potentially addictive painkiller, these workouts are designed to heal the root cause of the pain and therefore get rid of it for good. Painkillers are designed to block or drown the pain message, not cure the cause of the pain. Correct exercises will heal the cause.

**Repair damage:** The body is designed to heal itself. When the mechanics are working in harmony, your body can repair most existing damage. The Fast Track plan rebalances your body's mechanics, strengthening and increasing the flexibility of your muscles, improving the pliability of your ligaments, and hydrating and lubricating your fascia.

**Break the phantom pain loop:** Learning to work in a pain-free mode helps break the phantom pain loop, healing both the neurological *and* the real physical cause of pain. The last thing we want to do is trigger a pain loop by exacerbating an existing pain sensitivity.

**Heal chronic pain:** The Starter Workout is a great place to begin if you are in chronic pain. The aim is to learn how to find and then stay in a pain-free zone while still exercising. Remember, the exercises, the actual movements, are what heals you. Correct full-body exercises are your medication, but they work only if you do them in a pain-free mode. In some cases, remaining pain free might require hardly moving at all until you can move 100 percent pain free. Some people may take a few minutes, others a few days. Move until the pain starts and then return to the intensity where you were pain free. Use that intensity as your base point.

After living with chronic pain for so long, finding the pain-free sweet spot while exercising can be difficult. Once you figure out how to work in your pain-free zone, keep testing your pain limits. Try working a little harder until the pain kicks in. Then go back to the pain-free zone. Keep testing for new pain limits so that you can safely readjust and expand your movements and intensity. It may take several days or a few weeks, but you will notice that as the days go by, you are capable of working harder and doing more of the sequence in a pain-free mode. When you are fully pain free, you will know the healing is done.

It took me several years after starting this program to be 100 percent pain free after a lifetime of chronic pain. But for probably ten years now I have been 100 percent pain free, and let me tell you, it makes me feel young and alive! I have worked with many people who have suffered horrendous pain for decades. Until they tried this approach, they'd accepted their pain as their personal cross to bear. It's a sad fact of life, but many people can hardly move without being in pain. Even the smallest movement of an arm or leg can shoot pain throughout their body. If you are one of these people, try finding that pain-free zone—even if your movements are imperceptible to the naked eye. Most of the time, it is in this imperceptible place of almost zero movement that the miracle of healing begins. That sweet spot of zero pain will begin to widen, and before you realize what has happened, you'll be doing the whole workout with no pain. By the end of these 30 days, your pain might have disappeared forever—and you'll never have to tolerate it again.

# CHAPTER 5

WAY 5
# USE RELAXATION TO STRENGTHEN

Yes, you read that correctly. *Relaxation* is the way to increase your strength and reverse your age. It's a bit of a brain twister, I know. Relax to grow stronger? At first glance, this statement seems to be an oxymoron. But through my research and work with clients, I've learned that it is an absolutely astonishing way to rapidly increase strength and grow younger.

Did you know that overtraining is as damaging to your health as being sedentary? It's not a message people want to hear, especially those in the fitness world. Even though it's a controversial position, over these past years I have been outspoken in my condemnation of the overtrained body. As a former professional ballet dancer, I have experienced firsthand the negative impact of overtraining on the body. In addition to my own experience, the decades I've spent teaching hundreds of world-class athletes and dedicated weekend warriors how to get out of pain have reinforced my position.

People are open to hearing about the health damage a sedentary lifestyle does to the body—rapid aging, muscle weakness, disease, and chronic pain—but nobody wants to be told that their favorite training regimen or sport may be causing them to age rapidly. Many people are so deeply invested in their hard-core training and the belief that it will help them to relieve stress or achieve peak performance that they simply do not want to hear that they are actually doing damage to their body.

Many clients, especially the Type A hard chargers, want me to train them as hard as possible, firm in the faith that only hard work brings good results. They brag about how many sit-ups, push-ups, and chin-ups they can do. But I'm not impressed; instead I cringe, knowing the harm they are doing to their muscles, bones, and connective tissue. The ones who resist my gentle relaxation-based approach and go back to the "no pain, no gain" training often end up pushing themselves so hard that they tear a tendon, rip a ligament, or blow a rotator cuff, often needing surgical treatment to replace a knee or reattach a ligament. I warned them! So many people who train hard end up getting badly injured, putting an end to their extreme training. They usually come back to me, tail between their legs, with a greater willingness to try rebuilding their body my way. Please take this opportunity to make your life easier—and better—by learning from other people's mistakes instead of making the same ones yourself.

The fact that overtraining causes premature aging shouldn't be a total surprise. Overtraining causes intense stress on the body. Chronic stress can cause more than just musculoskeletal injuries. It can lead to inflammation, digestive issues, chronic fatigue, insomnia, and mood changes. A stressed body is not youthful or vibrant.

What is surprising is that relaxation, the opposite of overtraining, is an extremely powerful and safe *strengthening* technique. In other words, there is more than one way to gain strength. And the beauty of using relaxation to strengthen is that it doesn't lead to injuries and damage; it is healing and age-reversing. This is why my favorite new motto is "Relaxation is the new strengthening."

It took me a while to appreciate the power of relaxation. For years as an instructor, I'd use verbal corrections to try to get my students to do the Essentrics exercises correctly. I'd repeat the same correction over and over again, like "bend your elbow" or "bend your knee," but many people just never seemed to be able to physically do what I was saying. Their elbow or knee was sort of locked in a permanent barely bent position. How could this be? People were locked in these robotic-looking bodies, and for the longest time I could not figure out how to liberate their joints from their stiff movements.

Once I realized the issue was neurological—not due to the physiology of their muscles or connective tissue—I could finally help to unlock their stiffness. I had been focusing on the wrong cause of stiffness. It wasn't that people didn't understand my correction—they were simply incapable of bending because their nervous system didn't know how to release the tension in their muscles. They didn't know how to relax!

By looking beyond the muscles and directly at the nervous system, I discovered the hidden explanation for why so many people look robotic in their movements. If you can't release muscle tension, you can't move your joints smoothly through their full range of motion. This explained to me why so many people's muscles are in a permanent state of semi-contraction or semi-tension. The gracefulness of a ballet dancer's movements comes from his or her ability to fully bend or straighten a limb. When you can do neither completely, your body exhibits jerky, robotic movements.

## A BODY AS STIFF AS HARD PLASTIC

Chronically tense or contracted muscles waste energy and raise our blood pressure. A constant state of tension impedes the efficient circulation of blood, thus reducing the delivery of oxygen and other nutrients to the muscles. Poor circulation also limits the flushing action of the interstitium to rid the body of the waste products, leaving us tired, achy, and sore. Immobility causes muscles to weaken and atrophy. The fascia surrounding these muscles slowly congeals until it forms a rigid sleeve. The remolded fascia locks the muscle down and prevents movement. When this happens, the body starts to appear as stiff as hard plastic. Relaxation stops and reverses this negative chain reaction.

We are so accustomed to building strength through rough, harsh movements that contract and create tension in our muscles and joints. As a result, trillions of our muscle fibers forget how to relax when we move. Yet some of the greatest strength is found in elongated, relaxed muscles. Picture a cheetah running, muscles long and sinewy, offering immense speed and power to the animal. Its muscles are not contracted and tense, but lengthened with explosive power, not straining at all. If cheetahs did contract their muscles, they would lose their speed and power. Picture a ballet dancer flying through the air, legs apart, at incredible speed and then rapidly shifting direction to perform an even more explosive leap. The immensely strong muscles of the cheetah and the ballet dancer are released to permit the massive explosive movements.

Healthy muscle cells are designed to move effortlessly, in a nanosecond, sliding in and out of their telescope-type shaft as they either contract or lengthen. When we don't straighten or bend our joints to their full extension or flexion, the muscle cells lose their ability to slide in and out of their shaft. The muscles are in effect being trained to hold the joints at a limited degree of flexion or extension; holding requires tension. The neurological system is being trained to lock the muscles in place. In time the brain literally forgets how to completely relax the joints to their full extension.

But you can help your brain to remember. Our brain, our master controller, is in charge of the tension in our muscles. Once you become aware of the tension and tightness in your joints, you can retrain your brain to release it. By bringing your attention and focus to the area of tension, you can "tell" your brain to relax and release the tension so that the limb can bend and lengthen fully. We have the ability to focus the brain on relaxing the muscles, commanding the tension to dissolve. It takes a little bit of mental effort to find the tension in any particular spot and then use a laser beam of concentration to force the tension to dissipate, but anyone can do it. Once you master the art of relaxation, you reset the control switch that had been set on "limited length." The blood starts to flow, the fascia loosens, your skin takes on a vibrant glow, and a youthful bounce returns to your movements. All this from relaxation.

And you can finally move.

## THE SCIENCE BEHIND "RELAXATION IS THE NEW STRENGTHENING"

According to a basic law of physics, the longer a lever is, the heavier the load it can lift. A seesaw is a lever in its simplest form: a long, rigid arm (like a board or a pole) that hinges on a pivot point called a fulcrum. The human body is full of levers of various lengths. There is one found at all 360 of our joints. A lever could be our arm, leg, or torso; a lever in the human body is any part that can bend, twist, turn, or lift. The fulcrum or pivot point is the point that allows movement, like the hinge of the seesaw. Your elbow is the pivot point for your arm, for example.

Our body works a little bit like a seesaw: For one part to move, the opposite part has to release it. As a child, you may have experienced being held up in the air at one end of the seesaw when the heavier person on the other end won't get off and let you down.

The 210 bones of our body are in a constant interplay; one side moves and the attached opposite side releases. This takes place at joints. If your muscles are held in a constant state of semi-tension, your joints cannot bend or straighten completely. This means that your muscles are also only half sliding in and out. Their movement is restricted.

Now remember that law of physics: the longer the lever, the heavier the load. Logically speaking, the heavier the load, the more the muscles have to work to lift that load. Lifting fifty pounds takes more strength than lifting ten pounds. If you can relax the muscles and fully extend the limbs, you can make your legs, arms, and torso longer levers, capable of lifting more weight. Simply by relaxing the tension, you can force your joints to extend to their full length and exponentially increase the strength of your muscles. *Relaxation is the new strengthening.* Try it as you do the Fast Track workouts. It really works.

## FAST TRACK WITH RELAXATION

Our muscles are created or designed to be strong well into our nineties. When you use relaxation in unison with the Fast Track exercise sequences, you can *have your cake and eat it, too.* These exercises will help you to:

Grow stronger: The more you relax, the farther you can bend, stretch, and reach, and your strength will exponentially increase. Just in case you need more convincing, a review of twenty studies that looked at the effects of the Fast Track type of eccentric exercise, published in the *British Journal of Sports*

*Medicine,* found that when compared with concentric exercise (in which muscles contract), eccentric exercise (in which muscles elongate) is clearly superior in improving muscle strength and mass.[10]

Access more muscles: Relaxation lengthens your load, which increases your ability to strengthen your muscles while allowing you to finally access muscles you've never exercised before. The human body is made up of many layers of muscle groups. The smallest muscles are closest to the center of our body, closest to the actual bones. The outer muscles are the largest, while muscles found closer to the center of the body are the smallest. Most fitness programs tend to focus on strengthening the larger muscles, as they are the biggest, strongest ones. This is because so many still believe that since we need the largest muscles to do the heavy lifting of the body, they are the most important muscles.

As the large muscles are being strengthened, the tiny inner muscles are overwhelmed and not given a chance to work. Over time they become weaker and lose their ability to do their job of supporting and stabilizing the joints. We end up with all kinds of joint damage and pain. In order to prevent this from happening, we need to strengthen the little, or micro, muscles. In order to do that, we must first play down the use of weight training to strengthen the largest outer muscles and put the emphasis on full-body strengthening.

Full-body strengthening is most effective when you release or relax the largest muscles into elongated movement as you do large full-body movements. (You will find these large sequences throughout every workout in this book.) As the macro muscles release, the micro or smaller muscles are forced to do their work of stabilizing and supporting the joints, becoming stronger in the process. The more you relax as you move, the easier it becomes to access and strengthen these muscles.

Due to their location close to the joints, the little muscles have control over how much you can bend and move. If the little ones shrink from disuse, they will limit your ability to move. You will feel stiff and old. The more capable you are of moving (bending, twisting, turning, stretching), the stronger you will become and the younger you will feel. So again, *relaxation is the new strengthening.*

Loosen up: We become robotic in our movements through poor body habits. Learning to relax while exercising takes a bit of practice, but once you get the hang of it, you'll see how wonderful it feels to do—and how great the results can be. Relaxation can transform an awkward, weak, stiff person into a graceful one quite rapidly. And it works for everyone, from novice exercisers all the way up to the most committed fitness professionals.

Strangely enough, relaxing your muscles requires a great deal of concentration, and you will find that moving the body at the same time as you are relaxing it takes even more work. Don't be surprised if you start to perspire just by relaxing. That's because you are using muscles that you've all but forgotten you have. By working in the relaxation mode, you are awakening and stimulating muscles that may have gone unused for so long that they have partially atrophied.

Throughout the Fast Track workouts are prompts and reminders to tap into the power of relaxation and focus your attention on releasing tension. The more you practice relaxation, the more natural and intuitive it will feel. You'll immediately recognize when a part of your body is tense and be able to release it.

At teacher-training workshops, I start by explaining the power of relaxation. Sounds like an easy first assignment, right? Well, I have rarely seen people sweat so hard as when a group of strong, vibrant instructors begin to learn to relax. It takes time and practice!

With these ideas in mind, I started experimenting with my students, spending a considerable amount of class time just on relaxation—getting them to relax their knees, their elbows, their shoulders, their backs, their necks, their fingers. By the end of these unconventional classes, everyone was bouncing off the walls with increased energy and strength. I would highly recommend that you try to teach your joints to relax prior to doing your workouts to get familiar with how it feels. As you do the warm-up movements, try your best to completely relax your shoulders, elbows, wrists, and fingers. If you are having trouble, try visualizing that you are boneless, nothing more than a rag doll. Watch yourself in a mirror to see if you are looking more graceful and less robotic. You will enjoy learning to relax because it feels so good. Once you master this technique, your body will automatically use your 650 muscles in everyday life. With the recruitment of the full musculature of your body, you will feel as if you've lost considerable weight because moving becomes easy.

I've since worked with hundreds of people on how to use relaxation as their new strengthening, and the results never fail to thrill everyone. Usually within one or two days of relaxation with the Fast Track workouts, people look years younger. It's shocking in a good way!

Since I have been using relaxation as my primary strengthening mode, I am stronger and more energetic than ever.

# CHAPTER 6

WAY 6

# CREATE A DAILY HABIT OF EXERCISE

All the information in this book is useless if you don't develop a habit of doing the exercises. Knowing how to rebalance your muscles, strengthen your bones, and hydrate your connective tissue won't do you any good if you don't do the exercises every day. We have found that the exponential benefits are so much greater when you do this program every day that we have decided to suggest that you try seven days a week rather than "as often as possible" or "five times a week." It goes without saying that any amount of exercising is better than none, but this book is about getting you on the Fast Track of aging backwards, so it would be unfair for me to suggest that you would get the same results if you opted for five days a week. That being said, if you can't exercise seven days a week, then do the best you can. You will get some results. The more often and more consistently you do the exercises, the better your results will be.

Our daily habits influence our lives, for better or for worse. "We are what we repeatedly do," wrote the American historian and philosopher Will Durant in 1926.

"Excellence, then, is not an act, but a habit." I am lucky in that the habit of daily exercise has been a steadfast ally of mine since I enrolled in the National Ballet School of Canada at the age of ten.

A dancer's life is all about habits and routine. At the professional ballet boarding school I lived in as a young ballerina, they taught us to develop good eating habits to ensure we ate sufficient quantities of healthy food to supply enough energy without overeating and weight gain. Our daily routine was engineered so that when the ballet teacher arrived in the studio, we'd already warmed up, the ribbons on our ballet slippers were securely sewn so as not to rip off when we went on pointe, our tights and leotards were clean, and our hair was secured in a tight bun with not a hair out of place. If I'd had the habit of being late or sloppy, I would have been expelled and that would have been the end of my dreams of a dancing career.

As a professional ballerina, I faced an even greater pressure to be disciplined; the habits we created and routines we followed in school were essential in helping all us dancers withstand the rigors of a performer's life. As a performer, you have to be ready for curtain call. Getting my hair and makeup finished before curtain call took me three hours. Some dancers could do it in an hour, but I needed three hours because I have really thick hair and my eyes are difficult to make up. This long preparation required me to develop the habit of arriving two hours before everyone else. The habit of being disciplined has remained with me my entire life.

We tend to think of routines as a type of drudgery, but developing that routine to arrive three hours before call time *liberated* me. I never had to wonder or worry about when to go to the theater; I just went out of habit.

In hindsight, I realize how habits and constructive routines have allowed me to accomplish much more than I might have without them. The habit of knowing how long things take has helped me to juggle my present busy life of travel, teaching, writing, and creating new *Classical Stretch* television programs. I automatically slip into new habits that help me make the best use of my time to reach my goals.

Contemporary scientists tell us that habits become second nature through repetition.[11] They form the bedrock of everyday life. Chances are you don't really have to think about the weekday morning routine that gets you out of bed, showered, dressed, fed, and on the way to work—it's a practiced sequence of events that likely no longer requires any conscious effort to execute. Once they were established, these habits became the invisible assistants that allow us to focus on other things, including what we want to accomplish during the day. Each day, if we had to debate with ourselves the merits of brushing our teeth or the necessity of a shower, we'd never get anything done. By making basic hygiene an unconditional habit, we get going quickly and easily.

Once we accept the fact that daily upkeep of our bones, muscles, and connective tissue is just as important as our dental hygiene, then we will add them as part of our morning or evening habits.

## THE FAST TRACK HABIT

The Fast Track plan is designed to help you create a habit of daily exercise through repetition and rewards.

Commit for 30 days. Forming new habits can be challenging at first. It requires dedicated, conscious attention for a certain period of time in order to lay the neural grooves in your mind to make the new behavior feel normal, natural, and welcome. If you commit and force yourself for these 30 days, you'll have a much greater chance of creating a habit that will be significantly easier to keep for life.

Do it every day. Researchers have found that as much as 40 percent of our everyday activities tend to be repeated in the same location almost every day.[12] That's one of the reasons I believe you should do your program *every day*—not just three times a week, not just every other day, but *every day*. Our objective is to make your exercise routine just as automatic and nonnegotiable as brushing your teeth or making coffee—you don't just skip those on the weekends, do you? When you do it on a daily basis, your morning (evening) Fast Track workout will feel so instinctive and necessary that if you *don't* do it, you will feel like something is missing.

Clarify your "want to do." In his landmark book *The 7 Habits of Highly Effective People,* Stephen R. Covey defines a habit as the intersection of knowledge, skill, and desire. "Knowledge is the theoretical paradigm, the *what to do* and the *why,*" Covey writes. "Skill is the *how to do.* And desire is the motivation, the *want to do*. In order to make something a habit in our lives, we have to have all three."

You've already taken the first steps. You've recognized the need to change and to improve your self-care. You've acquired this book and opened its pages, beginning a learning process that can lead to a better you.

To make a habit you have to build a strong emotional foundation to support your habit; keep reminding yourself that doing these exercises on a daily basis will experientially improve every aspect of your life. You'll look better and feel better. Your relationships will improve because you'll be free of pain. You'll do your work with more energy and greater joy. Are you feeling better, stronger, younger? More energized, free of pain, healthier? Be very conscious of these benefits. Use these rewards as motivation to stick to the habit.

Visualize exactly how you would like your life to look in a year. Consider why full-body exercise is so important by reflecting on what you have learned about how to rejuvenate your body. Write a list of the most important reasons for doing this program, and use these reasons as your touchstone when you want to press the snooze button or watch another episode on Netflix. Fast Track with Essentrics first; the rest of life comes afterward.

**Make it fit your life.** The Fast Track plan boasts many features that allow you to turn it into a habit easier than you might think. You don't have to drive, cycle, or walk to the gym. Or participate in an hour-long class. (And other than what you paid for this book, it's free!) You can finish your sequences at home in as little as 20 to 30 minutes. You can do them in your pajamas without worrying about how you look. For some people, putting on workout clothes is a barrier, but at home you don't have to bother! Do the workouts in stretchy jeans. Heck, you can do them naked!

**Connect it to another habit.** Habits come in different forms and levels of intensity. Some people will not leave the breakfast table before checking the weather forecast, yet they'll skip putting the dirty dishes in the sink.

One of the most powerful ways to create a new habit is to anchor it to an existing one. Take the example of brushing your teeth: You likely (hopefully!) do it every day, without fail. Plan to do your daily exercise right after brushing your teeth. Tape a reminder to your toothbrush ("When I'm done with this, I will do my workout"). Here are a few other ideas:

- If you normally check email or social media while your spouse is showering in the morning, tell yourself: "When he/she gets in the shower, I start my workout."

- Get out of bed at the same time and do your workout before your coffee. Or connect it with your coffee routine: "While the pot is brewing, I will do my workout." As soon as you press *brew*, go into the living room and get it done.

- If you prefer to do your workout in the afternoon or evening, anchor it to your return home: "When I enter the house and take off my shoes, I do my workout." Then you can get it done before you even head to the kitchen or the couch.

**Remind yourself constantly.** As you are trying to establish the exercise habit, leave little reminder notes in key areas—next to your alarm clock, on the bathroom mirror, on the kitchen table. On every reminder note, reinforce your "want to do" reasons: "I work out after I brush my teeth to improve my flexibility," or "I work out while the coffee brews so I can have more energy and think more clearly all day." Leave notes for yourself in places where you are likely to be tempted off course—on the refrigerator, on the television, on the telephone.

**Tell yourself: "No excuses for 30 days."** There may be times when your resolve weakens and you think about skipping a day. Maybe you didn't have a great night's sleep; you can't find your favorite exercise gear; a friend telephoned wanting to chat. Don't get distracted. Remind yourself that you have committed to building this additional habit of self-care.

Don't get down on yourself if you fall off the wagon. After all, no one is perfect, and the pressure to be so can derail our best intentions. Instead, trick yourself into tapping your inner wellspring of willpower by pledging "no excuses for the next day." It may help to tell yourself that the Fast Track plan is a temporary habit—you're committing to it for only 30 days. Most of us can handle a 30-day commitment. When the first 30 days are over, ask yourself, "How do I feel?" Rather than thinking about doing Fast Track workouts as a lifelong daily habit (which may seem intimidating at first), think of doing them as a month-long streak. Chances are, once the 30-day plan is over, you will feel so fantastic that you'll want to continue forever!

**Do it in the morning.** Based on the thousands of emails and letters I've received, most people like to do their exercise routines in the morning. The most common reason I've heard is that they like to get it out of the way before getting on with the rest of life. Fair enough! And in the evening there are often distractions like dinner with friends, going to a movie, or being just plain exhausted from a day's work. According to Cedric Bryant, PhD, chief science officer with the American Council on Exercise in San Diego, "Research suggests in terms of performing a consistent exercise habit, individuals who exercise in the morning tend to do better" and have a better chance of sticking with the habit over the long term. But whatever time of day you choose, try to be consistent.[13]

Your body urgently needs daily exercise. Use the Fast Track plan to help you create a habit and make sure it happens. You have everything to gain and nothing to lose. The ultimate rewards at the end of this 30-day program are better health, better mobility, energy, and sharper cognition. You will have aged backwards.

# CHAPTER 7

# CHANGE YOUR LIFE FOREVER

## *Use the 6 Ways to Prevent and Reverse the Most Common Signs of Aging*

Aging doesn't really have an age, but it does have a signature—immobility! When we are young, we tend to view aging in the abstract, dimly aware that we are getting old. We don't really believe that aging will happen to us until a change in our body causes an interruption in our daily life. We can ignore stiffness for a long time. But stiffness is the precursor of immobility, and once we experience that—maybe we can no longer effortlessly dress ourselves, reach into higher or lower cupboards, or walk upstairs—the harsh realization hits: we're aging. Often, fear and anxiety about our future arrive, too. However, aging doesn't have to be feared.

With the Fast Track plan, you can consciously decide to age backwards. Even in your senior years, you can go back and change your body and thus reclaim your youth.

All you need to do is tap into the *miracle of movement*. Remember movement is the signature of youth and immobility the signature of aging.

I hope you're beginning to understand how the six ways of the Fast Track plan work together, reinforcing one another to reverse your aging process. Now let's look at ten of the most common complaints people have as they get older—and how Essentrics can help you fight each one.

Think of them the way we now know we should think of pain: as a signal that it's time to make a change! Whether you have all of these warning lights flashing right now, or just a few of them, the Fast Track exercises will give your body what it needs to turn them off. If you don't have any of these signs, that's wonderful! These exercises will keep it that way.

Whether these ten signs show up because you have misused your body or have had poor habits or they are the legacy of injuries or surgeries, you can reverse them and keep them away for good.


## POOR POSTURE

Nothing makes people look older than poor posture. However, it's not only about appearance. Poor posture has a direct negative effect on our health. A rounded back interferes with our ability to breathe deeply and to digest our food, and it even affects the health of our heart.

While poor posture has many basic causes, the most common is the most obvious: years of slouching. (See, Mom was right when she told us to stand up straight!) Over time, slouching deforms the muscles and connective tissue. When the shoulders droop forward, the muscles of the upper back become overstretched and weak from being in one consistent position. The fascia in these disused muscles slowly congeals, stiffening and virtually hardening. This congealing of the upper back is visible to the eye—you'll see no mobility in that region—but it is also easy to identify by touch. The upper back feels rigid and hard, with no muscle movement rippling under the skin.

In addition to a habit of slouching, hours spent bent over a computer or engaged in extreme weight training, which overbuilds the shoulder and back muscles, are also common causes of poor posture. For example, you may notice that people who do a lot of push-ups, chin-ups, and weight training tend to stoop forward and have really stiff upper backs.

Prevention: The best defense to combat poor posture is daily strengthening, mobility, and flexibility exercises of the full body, making sure to involve the muscles and the connective tissue equally. This requires slow movements that work the full range of motion of the shoulders, spine, hips, and legs.

> The use of free weights or any type of weight training is not recommended to reverse poor posture. Weights are often one of the *causes* of overbuilt, tight upper backs, as they shorten the muscles, leading to compressed joints.

Reversal: Poor posture is the sign of unbalanced muscles and congealed fascia. It will take time to rebalance those muscles and de-congeal glued fascia. Be patient. Muscles strengthen within days, but fascia takes months and sometimes years to de-congeal depending on how far back the congealed state developed. When stronger muscles like pectorals are strengthened with push-ups and weights, they pull the upper back into a rounded, poor posture.

To reverse this, first stop strength training the major muscles. You'll need to be patient as you give your back muscles time to strengthen as the pectorals release some of their dominance and open up.

Regular stretching, strengthening, and rebalancing exercises are the only way to reverse poor posture. (While you must do the entire Fast Track workout to get the benefit, exercises such as raising your arms above your head, side bends, and hamstring stretches are particularly helpful for reversing poor posture.) Some people see results rapidly, as early as within a week of starting. But realistically, severe poor posture caused from unbalanced, overbuilt, or weak muscles can take three to six months to reverse.

You wouldn't stop taking a course of antibiotics until it's complete, even if your symptoms have abated, would you? The same is true of these workouts! Don't stop doing the rebalancing exercises even after your posture improves. Your connective tissue has an excellent memory and will try to return to the poor posture configuration if you stop exercising. As the gentle exercises of the Fast Track plan become part of your daily life, you won't have to worry about the return of poor posture.

## POOR BALANCE

Losing our balance as we age is scary. There are many possible causes, such as changes in our peripheral vision or in the balance crystals in our ears. But poor balance most commonly results from poor skeletal alignment and weak muscles.

The traditional explanation for poor balance is that we lose balance reflexes with age. People say it's a natural consequence of aging. You won't be surprised to learn that I disagree: There's a great deal we can do to maintain good balance as we age.

Yes, it is true that we lose some balance reflexes, but the loss of nerve cells is caused by the "use it or lose it" principle, not aging. Poor alignment is a major cause of poor balance, and we know the causes of poor alignment (not standing flat on the soles of our feet, standing with our weight on the inside or outside of our feet or general muscular weakness). Having poor balance has little to do with aging but everything to do with poor alignment in the ways we stand, sit, and walk. Most people have trained their muscles and joints to be out of alignment.

Standing incorrectly on the soles of our feet is probably the number one way in which people destroy their alignment. Our feet are designed to be our foundation, and when the way we stand on our feet is off, the rest of the skeleton will be pulled out of alignment. When we roll our ankles inward or outward, the full weight of our body loads that side of the chain of muscles up our leg, overstressing those muscles, while the muscles along the opposite chain become overstretched and weak. This pulls the ankle, knee, and hip joints out of alignment, becoming the definition of an unbalanced body.

It's only logical that with these muscular imbalances from poor alignment we would become unstable on our legs as we age.

**Prevention:** Good balance requires standing flat on the soles of our feet, clean skeletal alignment, and strong, flexible, full-body muscles.

Practice standing on the *full* sole of your foot. This will require standing with your weight distributed from the heel to the full pad of the foot (where the toes join your sole). Imagine your feet rooted in the earth and experiment with slowly rolling your feet internally, then externally. Again, you want to spread the weight of the body evenly from the front pad of your foot to the heel pad, the center point being the middle of the arch of your feet. If you can't quite tell if you are inverting (rolling in) or everting (rolling out) your ankles, check the soles of the shoes you walk most in.

If you find a wedge shape worn in the heel of your shoes, this wedge shape will tell you which applies.

Practice keeping your feet planted in place as you shift your weight back and forth, adjusting your feet so the soles are flat on the ground. (Warning: Correct placement of your feet will feel uncomfortable for a few weeks as you are strengthening the weak muscles and stretching the overstrengthened contracted ones.)

Children should be trained to stand correctly on the full soles of their feet. We could all have perfect balance if we learned perfect foot alignment in our childhood and maintained it thereafter. This is best learned when a baby is starting to walk through the age of three. Keep your toddlers barefoot as much as possible throughout their day, giving their arches and feet a chance to develop naturally. This will save them from suffering from poor alignment and joint problems as they age.

**Reversal:** First, learn to stand on the full soles of your feet. That is easier said than done, as you probably won't have sufficient strength or flexibility to maintain the sole of your foot flat on the floor for longer than a few seconds. We were all born with the ability to stand on the soles of our feet; we just didn't cultivate it over time. It is one of the most important adjustments you can make while doing this program, so keep working at it until you succeed.

After you have mastered standing on the full sole of your foot, begin to retrain and rebalance the muscles to support your joints in perfect alignment through your ankles, knees, hips, and spine. If your joints are poorly aligned—and those of most people are—you will find that standing on the soles of your feet is difficult, uncomfortable, and awkward at first. And exhausting! You probably won't like how it feels for a few weeks, but be patient, as good sole alignment will ultimately change your life. This is because your unbalanced muscles are trying to pull you back into your old comfortable poor alignment. You will be having a constant tug-of-war with your muscles whenever you walk and stand, but you will win. Stay mindful of your feet and correct them when you feel them slipping into their old ways.

In the Starter Workout and the Fast Track Core Workouts, you'll find many exercises for the feet. Again, with daily exercise you will reap the rewards of improved balance as your feet alignment improves.

# IT'S NEVER TOO LATE TO
# FIND YOUR BALANCE

A sixty-five-year-old friend of mine recently started complaining of stiffness and increasingly frequent bouts of mild to medium pain in her right ankle. She couldn't flex her right foot and she felt a tightness in her right Achilles tendon that often traveled up into her leg muscles. In order to avoid aggravating her right ankle, she compensated by using her left leg more.

When orthopedic specialists viewed an X-ray, they found floating bone fragments and other evidence of an old trauma near the right ankle joint. It took my friend some time to link her ankle problem with a skydiving mishap from *thirty-eight years earlier.* She had landed badly and suffered a bad break of her *left* ankle and minor trauma to the right ankle. They put her left leg in a full cast for about three months, but virtually ignored her twisted but not broken right one. (Orthopedic treatments were much different then!) Her left ankle healed "stronger than ever," but the right one never fully healed. As my friend approached her sixties, she gained weight, increasing the stress on all of her joints. Her increased weight caused pain in her right ankle, and thankfully she listened to it.

This story has a happy ending. She is now aware that she needs to nurture her right ankle by ensuring her daily routine includes exercises that focus on ankles and feet. With daily Essentrics workouts, she rebooted the muscle chains in her right leg so they are free-flowing, the pain is gone, and she no longer favors one leg over the other. Once her body was rebalanced, the thirty-eight-year-old injury finally healed. She doesn't worry any longer about being off-balance and falling.

## GENERAL STIFFNESS AND LACK OF SUPPLENESS

One of the major complaints of aging is a general feeling of stiffness. It often manifests as an inability to pull a sweater over the head or get in and out of a car. The cause of most stiffness is usually from either too much or too little activity.

Walking doesn't solve the problem of full-body atrophy. Walking is great for fresh-air exercise and for the few muscles the body uses to do it. The motion of walking is performed by a pendulum action of the leg swinging in the hip, mostly activated by momentum and not muscle activity. So it is not a serious fitness program (although it can be useful if it is done rapidly and preferably up and down hills).

A lack of general activity causes the interstitium (the liquid layers within the fascia sheets) to slowly congeal and harden, becoming a stiff sleeve around your muscles. Remember, the interstitium should act like an oily lubricant between the layers of the fascia, allowing the fascia layers to slip and slide over one another. When the fascia has the ability to stretch and retract, then the muscles the fascia surrounds can also stretch and contract. When inactivity glues the interstitium together, then the fascia bag surrounding the muscles cannot move, which directly affects the muscles encased within the fascia. Congealing fascia is one reason why we feel stiff! But don't worry, there is a wide range between slightly gummy and totally hardened connective tissue. Most people are usually in the beginning stages of congealing, where they feel a slight stiffness but are still fully capable of sitting, standing, and walking. The stiffness is slightly limiting but easily reversible with a good stretching workout or therapeutic massage. The longer you have been inactive, the more the fascia will have hardened. This happens only after years and years of inactivity. At that point, walking, sitting, and standing are extremely difficult to do and the fascia may have become so dehydrated that it is brittle and easily tears.

The potential danger of extreme congealed fascia underscores the need to do daily stretches to maintain the slipping and sliding action between the layers. Daily full-body stretching prevents us from getting caught in a vicious cycle of muscle inactivity leading to more fascia congealing, leading to stiffness, leading to more muscle atrophy . . . You get the general idea!

Prevention: You can prevent this from happening only by doing regular—preferably daily—full-body gentle mobility and stretching exercises. As long as you move every muscle in your body at least once a day, no fascia will congeal and your muscles will not become stiff.

**Reversal:** Reversing congealed fascia and stiff atrophied muscles must be done slowly, carefully, and daily, with gentle mobility and stretching exercises. The human body is a self-healing machine that (in most circumstances) will heal itself when given half a chance. The gumminess is designed to loosen up and return to a healthy hydrated state if we introduce careful, slow stretching and mobility exercises. It takes time, but I've seen hundreds of people reverse what felt to the touch like solid packs of hardened connective tissue in their hunched backs, finally becoming capable of moving their upper backs totally freely. It takes time, years, but it's worth the effort.

A note for the very stiff: All the workouts in this book are designed to reverse congealed fascia; however, they are also strengthening. If you self-describe as very stiff, stick with the Starter Workout or the standing and chair portions of the Core Workouts (Part One) until your body doesn't feel uncomfortably stiff. Once you have loosened up, then try the strengthening floor exercises in the Core Workouts (Part Two). The strengthening floor exercises are more contracting and will counteract the benefits of stretching for you.

## CHRONIC PAIN

Chronic pain impacts more people than heart disease, diabetes, and cancer combined. In the era of rampant opioid abuse and overdose, addressing chronic pain without pharmaceutical drugs may actually save your life![14]

There are two types of pain: acute and chronic pain.

Acute pain comes on suddenly, and its cause is usually easily identifiable—a broken bone, surgery, an accident, or cancer. We know we are in acute pain, and it usually goes away within days with medical intervention.

Chronic pain is pain that has lasted longer than three months. It may have started as a minor irritant and, years later, developed into full-blown chronic pain. Further complicating the diagnosis of chronic pain is that we all have a different level of tolerance to pain. Ironically, people who have a very low pain tolerance will be healthier than those who can endure severe pain. People who can't endure pain will try to heal as quickly as possible, whereas people with a high pain tolerance will put up with it for decades. The high-tolerance people are usually athletes like boxers, ballet dancers, and football players.

When pain isn't fully resolved after an injury, surgery, or illness is declared healed by medical professionals, the pain is telling us that something is still wrong—*even if a doctor says our injury is healed.* The doctor may have finished his or her portion of the job of healing us, but we are responsible for the rest of our rehabilitation. Many people simply don't know how to go about self-rehabilitation. When in doubt, remember the mantra *movement is medicine!* The more you move and move wisely, gently with rehabilitation in mind, the faster you will heal.

Chronic pain is often caused by an unbalanced musculature due to repetitive motion at work, while playing sports or doing fitness activities, or from bad standing and walking habits. Repetitive motion in many sports like golf, baseball, swimming, and running will unbalance the musculature. Repetitive motion in fitness regimens—walking on a treadmill, pulling on weights, doing sun salutations in yoga, riding on a stationary bike—unbalances your body. Repetitive motion strengthens the muscles that are required to do the repetitive motion, leaving the other muscles of your body out of the equation. If you do such activities regularly, you are destined to unbalance your muscles. But you don't have to be athletic to become unbalanced; it seems just being alive is cause enough.

Most chronic pain is rooted in unbalanced muscles, which create poorly aligned joints. Even if you don't know the source—and don't waste too much of your time trying to solve the mystery of *how* you became unbalanced—now is the time to correct it by rebalancing your muscles and realigning your joints.

**Prevention and Reversal:** The only way to prevent and reverse chronic pain is to do rebalancing and realigning exercises daily. The Fast Track workouts are highly efficient at rebalancing because they include all 650 muscles. Any workout that misses any muscles cannot be considered a rebalancing program. As we know, muscle cells are tubular in shape, using a telescope-like action of contracting and extending as muscles shorten and lengthen. The fastest way to reverse the pain from unbalanced muscles is to do gentle full-body flexibility and mobility movements to fully restore the stretching and shrinking action within all the trillions of muscle cells that make up our 650 muscles. When the telescope-like sliding inside the cells is restored/rehabilitated, your body will be fully balanced and you will feel like you lost a hundred pounds. You will know when that happens because you will be pain free and will move easily.

All the workouts in this book are full-body rebalancing and realigning.

# DON'T RUN AWAY FROM YOUR PAIN

Faye, in her early fifties, enrolled in an Essentrics teacher-training course that spanned several days. She had a type A personality, no question about it. She'd just retired from a very successful but stressful career in a field dominated by men, one that required extreme physical strength and excessive travel. Her strength was no problem. She'd been a sportswoman all her life, excelling in individual and team sports. But her sporting activities didn't come without many severe injuries. Starting in her college years, she'd suffered from concussions, broken bones, and multiple torn and sprained muscles and ligaments. She never complained to her team coaches or companions, as she didn't want to look like a wimp. She was always trying to prove that she was up to anything. Because she didn't complain, she didn't take time off to completely heal. She just soldiered on until finally one day her body actually froze up.

She slowly worked her way back to some degree of mobility; however, by then chronic pain had overtaken every cell in her body. She had never considered that the many injuries she had endured might be the source of her chronic pain. The expression of pain on her face told the whole story. She couldn't hide it from anyone who cared to look. The deep crevices etched into her face alerted me that something was seriously wrong with her body.

During her first class, I quizzed Faye about where she felt pain. She denied having any. (Her drawn face said otherwise.) She was annoyed with me for invading her privacy (that's my job), but I persisted and she finally told her story. She didn't know what it was like *not* to be in pain, so she had come to accept pain as normal. Yet when she finally let her guard down, she recognized that actually her pain level was off the charts all the time.

To begin the process of freeing herself from pain, she first had to bring it into her awareness before she could learn how to let it go.

The first thing I did was have her stand in a comfortable stance and start focusing on relaxing one muscle at a time. Like self-hypnosis. Once she was fully relaxed, she was capable of just standing still, not moving, with zero pain.

However, due to the extremity of her situation, if she even moved an inch the pain shot through her body.

We went through a very, *very* slow process of elimination, trying to find out what was still a real injury and what was phantom pain. When someone is accustomed to extreme pain, they can suffer just as much from phantom pain as from real pain. The first thing I had to do was get rid of her phantom pain so I could get down to fixing the parts of her body that were still showing signs of inflammation (real pain).

The trick to getting rid of phantom pain is to move a tiny bit right up until a sharp pain hits and then stop at that point and wait patiently till the pain goes away. Then try again. Repeat that over and over again. When you arrive at the level or place where the pain does not go away, then you know you've found the actual place of injury.

Faye spent about six hours the first day moving almost imperceptibly, raising her arms, moving her legs, and bending her knees to identify the pain, and then relaxing, to make the pain go away. At the start of the day her arms were in pain even as they hung at her side. By the end of the day she could lift her arms slightly above her shoulder with zero pain. That was the first time in decades when she wasn't in absolute pain.

Faye had started to identify and then switch the phantom pain loop off. Phantom pain loop happens when the self-protection mechanism gets its wires mixed up. Faye moved very slowly so the brain had a chance to identify the places where there were no injuries. Thus one inch at a time the loop got reprogrammed until we found the real injuries.

Faye was very angry with me because I wouldn't let her have fun exercising with the rest of the class. The next morning she told the group that when she'd returned to her hotel that evening she was fuming about all the time and money she'd spent to travel to learn a fitness program, only to spend the entire day trying to relax. But something miraculous happened to her. She was standing in front of us looking like a completely different woman. Her face was relaxed and glowing and she looked about twenty years younger. She told us that her anger pushed her into "an emotional meltdown," where she spent much of the night crying as she realized how impactful those injuries had been. She'd spent her life trying to make her coach, her teammates, and her three ex-husbands happy. She had forgotten to care for herself.

As it happened, Faye would go on to heal those old injuries in the following weeks. But that would not—could not—have happened if she hadn't relaxed and rebalanced her body.

Faye's type A personality had been the source of her success in the work-place, on the soccer field, and on the ski slopes, but it worked against her when it told her to ignore pain messages. This experience taught Faye that admitting to her pain was not weakness. Only by facing her pain could she let it go and truly heal.

## FINGER AND HAND STIFFNESS

Finger and hand stiffness shows up when we try to do simple activities: when our grip weakens, making us drop things, or when we are incapable of opening a lid on a jar. When we have arthritic hands, we feel insecure driving a car and have difficulty buttoning clothes, tying shoelaces, sewing, or cooking with ease. As well as being one of the most common signs of aging, arthritic hands interfere with our living an independent life. Unfortunately, very few people realize this condition can be reversed with specific strengthening and flexibility exercises for the hands.

Our hands have 27 bones—a total of 54 between the two. Now consider that the human body has only 210 bones; more than 25 percent of all the bones and joints in your body are in your hands! The hands are primarily made up of bones, ligaments, and tendons, with very few muscles. Most of the muscles that animate our fingers and hands are actually in the lower arm.

The most common causes of finger and hand stiffness are rheumatoid arthritis or osteoarthritis. The third runner-up is repetitive motion injuries (such as carpal tunnel syndrome).[15] Most arthritis begins due to inactivity of the fingers, wrists, and hands. If your daily life requires you to use your fingers only a little (type, cut food, open a door), then the use-it-or-lose-it syndrome kicks in, resulting in shrinkage and atrophy!

When you don't use your hands, the muscles, tendons, and fascia of your arms will become dehydrated, dry, and weak, leading to immobility, tightness, atrophy, and joint compression. That atrophy will cause the joints of your hands to pull together, leading to inflammation, degradation of the joints, and arthritis.

Prevention: If you don't use your hands in your job or daily life activities (like gardening or doing laundry by hand or hand-sewing), then you must do exercises specifically aimed at fully stretching and strengthening the fingers and wrists. To prevent hand and finger arthritis and immobility, the finger muscles, ligaments, and tendons need to be exercised every day with daily *pliability* exercises—not stretching. These are deliberate movements that exercise all of the joints of the fingers with slow, deliberate movements that are not trying to increase the actual flexibility of the tissue but the mobility of the joint action.

In order to protect the weblike integrity of the ligaments, you must prevent stretching the fingers at all costs! To do that, you must focus on bending the joint, not pulling it. Avoid hand weights, as they shorten the muscles, increase the likelihood of arthritis by compressing the joints, and make bending even more difficult. The safest method of increasing mobility and pliability of your fingers is to simply open and close your hands from fist to open palm, and when your hands are open, try to spread your fingers as far apart as possible.

These simple finger exercises almost always prevent any tightness and arthritis. As your hand and finger strength increases, so will your finger mobility.

Reversal: When fingers and hands are in chronic pain, do slow, deliberate hand and finger exercises as found in the workouts. You can do these simple exercises as often as you want, even every hour for a few minutes at a time. To prevent injuring the ligaments, never force your fingers to spread apart or stretch more than they are capable of doing on their own. Know that each time you do your exercises, you will be hydrating the connective tissue. It takes time to rehydrate ligaments, so be patient. Keep doing your finger exercises, and over time you will see improvement.

## FEET AND ANKLE ISSUES

Losing the ability to wiggle our toes or flex our ankles leads to several undesirable signs of aging. The worst is finding ourselves to be unsteady on our feet, and another is taking shorter strides as we walk.

Our feet house 28 bones, for a total of 56 between them. For those keeping track, that's another 25 percent of your total skeletal system—leaving only 100 bones for the rest of your body! This should show you the extreme importance of feet and hands in the body. Almost all of the most important activities in our body include either the feet or the hands or both! Think about it. Eating, standing, walking, bathing, dressing, typing, driving, running, climbing—all need these valuable appendages. Yet we give very little thought to keeping them in tip-top shape. With a minimum amount of exercise, they can be kept in excellent working order throughout a long life. If we consider how important they are to our daily life, it's odd to realize that most people barely *use* their feet and toes, including athletes. This is because we keep shoes on all day, when we're participating in sports and fitness and even at home. As a result, our toes and feet slowly suffer from the use-it-or-lose-it syndrome.

We wear shoes to protect our feet from damage, which makes sense, but we must learn to go barefoot as much as possible at home and outside where it is safe, as on grass or a sandy beach! Encasing our feet in some sort of supportive footwear is like putting the foot in a cast or brace. If you've ever had a broken limb put in a cast for a few weeks, you'll notice how shrunken your muscles are when you take the cast off. We need to use our feet and take off our footwear as often as possible to maintain strong, vibrant, healthy, pain-free feet and calves.

Once we pass forty-five, one in four of us will struggle with foot pain, and one in six of us will have ankle pain.[16] And one of the most common causes of complaint about the feet is bunions, which are very much caused by poor alignment of the foot and little to no feet and toe strength and flexibility.

As with your hands, feet are made up primarily of bones, ligaments, and tendons; there are relatively few muscles in the actual foot. The muscles that animate your toes and soles of your feet are mostly found in your lower leg—the calf and shins.

Movement is as essential for our feet as it is for every other part of our body. If we don't wiggle our toes or flex and point our feet, the muscles, ligaments, and tendons will shrink, congeal, and harden. The result is stiff, immobile toes, ankles, calves, and shins! Remember that your calves and shins are the muscles that move your feet, so when we don't move the feet, we are also not moving the muscles that animate them.

Tightness is a signal that the muscles are shortening and perhaps even atrophying. Shrinking pulls the joints together, leading to inflammation, degradation of the joints, and eventually arthritis. Tight, stiff, painful distorted toes and feet are very, very common.

There are many types of foot pain. Plantar fasciitis, shin splints, and arthritis are the most common, and they can all be relieved with gentle correct movement. Remember that the cause of much foot pain is immobility, so the logical and correct remedy is mobility.

Prevention: Preventing foot pain is really quite easy—you just need five minutes of foot exercises that move the muscles, ligaments, and tendons every day. If you exercise your toes and ankles daily, they will never suffer from stiffness or arthritis. I've seen people in their mid-eighties with the feet of twenty-year-olds simply from having done regular footwork.

In addition to regular exercise, correct alignment of your feet is essential to being pain free. Alignment of the feet is the most ignored and misunderstood feature of the human body. I had never heard of foot alignment until I was trained in it by Dr. Bradley Bosick from Denver. He showed me how to find foot alignment by drawing a plumb line from your shinbone through the arch of the foot. (As you are doing the exercises in this book, use a mirror to check your foot alignment.) Make sure that you are standing flat on the sole of your foot with your weight evenly distributed across the entire sole and not shifted to either the inside or the outside of your foot.

Reversal: Chronic pain in your toes, feet, or Achilles tendon is caused by poor mechanics and can be relieved with correct exercises. The mini-workouts (page 347) offer easy-to-do calf, toe, and ankle exercises. Do these simple exercises as often as you want. Make a habit of constantly doing these movements while watching TV, reading, lying in bed, standing or sitting on the bus, or standing in a grocery line. Become a foot-fidgeter! Move, move, move those toes, feet, and ankles. Bend and straighten your knees to stretch the calf and shins, and lift and lower the heel to strengthen the alignment of the connective tissue.

I do toe, feet, calf, and shin movements all day long. I may look silly, but I feel great. You might worry that people will look at you and think you're weird. But rarely does anyone pay any attention.

# A WORD OF WARNING

When working with your Achilles tendon, *never* try to stretch the tendon. Simply bend and flex the ankle to increase the pliability. Many people overstretch their Achilles tendon by hanging their heels over a stair while dropping their weight downward. This will cause irreparable damage to the fibrous web of the connective tissue, ultimately weakening its natural dynamic rebound action. There are many safe foot exercises in these workouts that will safely increase the mobility of your Achilles tendon without fear of damage.

## UNEXPLAINED WEIGHT GAIN AND DIMINISHED ENERGY

No one is debating that the obesity epidemic is a problem in our country—and, increasingly, around the world. If trends continue, according to a Harvard study, by 2030 an estimated 38 percent of the world's adult population will be overweight and another 20 percent will be obese. In the United States, the most dire projections based on earlier trends point to more than 85 percent of adults being overweight or obese by 2030.[17]

Clearly, gaining weight is extremely easy to do in this country. I'm not a nutritionist, so I won't give nutritional advice. What I do know is the direct relationship between exercising and weight gain or loss.

Every one of the tens of trillions of muscle cells must be moved daily to prevent muscle cell atrophy. When muscle cells shrink and atrophy, with them go the mitochondria, which are the calorie-burning, energy-producing furnaces of our body. The mitochondria control our weight by burning calories, but if they disappear along with atrophied muscles, the mechanism to burn calories is lost. The excess weight makes us slow down even further, and we get into a perfect loop of unnecessary pain and aging. This is often explained as a slowing down of the metabolism, but the metabolism is slowing down only because we've lost some of our calorie-burning furnaces. The solution to this issue is to prevent atrophy by moving every one of our 650 muscles. The most efficient way to do that is in a full-body Fast Track workout.

Prevention: A regular full-body workout is the only way to prevent muscle atrophy (and the loss of mitochondria). Make sure it's a full-body one that actually engages all of your 650 muscles. To keep all of your muscles alive and fired up, you must twist, turn, bend, and reach on all the natural planes of the body.

If you analyze different fitness methods, you will notice that few involve the full body even when they claim to be full-body activities. A treadmill uses only a limited number of lower body muscles as you walk repetitively on the platform. Weight-training equipment is designed to repetitively train specific muscles. The repetitive action of a golf swing uses the same muscle over and over again, unbalancing the full body. The repetitive swing action of the legs and arms in walking uses a great deal of momentum and not too many muscles unless you walk rapidly up and down hills. Only a workout that engages the micro and macro muscles of all of the body is a full-body workout, one that is capable of activating the mitochondria all over the body to burn calories to help maintain a stable weight.

The Fast Track workouts in this book will stimulate your full body, safely activating your mitochondria with zero-impact aerobic movements. The gentleness and the limited length of the workouts contradict everything we've been told about exercising for weight loss. However, through testimonials from tens of thousands of clients, we've seen the weight loss that results from doing a full-body workout.

Reversal: Muscles are made up of tens of thousands of cells. Daily full-body exercise, starting today, is your secret weapon to rebooting the powerful calorie-burning mitochondrial furnaces in your muscle cells.

Don't worry if you have experienced some muscle cell atrophy. In most cases it can be reversed. It takes time to reverse, but as long as the muscle is still alive, it can be rebuilt. Only if a muscle has totally atrophied can it not be resuscitated. (All the more reason to get started now!)

You must exercise while dieting to maintain full muscle mass during a calorie-reduction period. When you diet and don't exercise, the mitochondria in your muscle cells will use muscle protein as a source of fuel to burn, cannibalizing the cells. You will lose weight, but from all the wrong places. Instead of burning fat, you will burn muscle protein cells, shrinking the size of your muscle. Initially you'll be thrilled to see your weight loss when you stand on the scale, but your joy will be short lived when you go off your diet and notice the pounds returning and even more packing on. When you lost muscle weight, you lost the mitochondria in the muscles. You are left with the same inflammatory fat tissue as before. This cannibalizing will cause immediate weight gain when you return to eating normally because you'll have fewer remaining mitochondria with which to burn calories.

Exercising while dieting, using your muscles, prevents the mitochondria from cannibalizing themselves. Rather, the mitochondria are asking for food and the body has to search outside of the muscle cell to find it, tapping into the fat reserves for the fuel. Exercising as you diet will prevent the yo-yo cycle of weight loss followed by weight gain that happens as you are dieting.

Bear in mind, with so many complicating factors, exercise is only one piece of the weight control story. But it's a major piece that you can do something about.

## HIP AND KNEE PAIN

Hip and knee replacement procedures are some of the fastest-growing surgeries in medicine. Each year for the past two decades, the number of these surgeries has increased by more than 100 percent. The actual procedure has been perfected to the point where patients often return home the same day of surgery. Most patients are very satisfied by their outcome. This is great until you factor into the equation the years of chronic pain leading up to hip or knee surgery. During this period any and every activity is accompanied by torturous pain. I'd like to stop the damage from happening in the first place. And it can be done with decompressing stretching and strengthening exercises that are designed to stop the joints from squeezing together by pulling them apart. These simple exercises, if done on a daily basis, will eliminate joint damage entirely.

Hip and knee trouble begin as the muscles shorten (caused by either a sedentary life or impact sports like running and weight training), pulling the joints tightly together, creating a type of vise grip, damaging the cartilage and glassy surface of the joint. Eventually the cartilage and surface of the joint are worn away—causing the tremendous pain of bone-on-bone contact. Most likely you will require a joint replacement. The hip and knee joints are capable of absorbing a tremendous amount of impact from daily life activities, but they cannot absorb impact if they have been compressed.

It's a scientific fact that joints are designed to last our full lifetime, damage free—as long as we take care of them. However, they're not designed to be permanently compressed and to withstand extreme stress or impact over a prolonged period of time—what I call "joint abuse."[18] This joint abuse leads to extreme pain and eventually results in more than a million knee and hip replacements every year in America.

Joint abuse comes in many forms. The most common ones are weak muscles, excess weight, and extreme exercise. So it's not surprising that joint replacements are most common in semi-sedentary people, the overweight population, and athletes (sports that involve excessive running, aerobics, or weight training). All these populations have shortened muscles and compressed joints.

As a former professional ballet dancer and an aerobics instructor, I am speaking from both personal experience as well as an evidence-based understanding of the damage extreme activities can do to joints. Luckily for me, I stopped doing intense impact training before my joints became permanently damaged. And thankfully, at the age of sixty-nine, I have been 100 percent pain free for many years—as have many of my older students.

The sad irony is that many people who engage in extreme exercise do it in the belief that it will keep them young. They are blissfully unaware that they are actually exacerbating the speed of their aging process.

## EXCESS WEIGHT AND JOINT PAIN

Picture your joints as the suspension in your car. Every brand of car is designed to support a specific weight load. If you regularly overload the car, the suspension will be become damaged. Gaining excess weight overloads your joints, damaging them. Any movement you do puts additional weight on them, potentially damaging them further.

Prevention: There are three things you can do to prevent knee and hip pain:

1. Keep your weight down.
2. Do regular full-body stretching and strengthening exercises.
3. Avoid extreme sports and high impact activities after age forty-five.

**Reversal:** As you do these daily strengthening and stretching exercises, make sure that you remain in a pain-free mode at all times. Thus you will not cause any further damage as you are decompressing your joints. Avoid all of the activities that will compress your joints like running, spinning, and heavy weight training. It takes time to be completely out of pain. However, once you are, you can slowly return to all of the activities you previously enjoyed with one exception: The moment you find the pain returning, stop until you have rebooted the muscles with the full-body decompressing stretches in this book. If you don't stop when you are in pain, you will find yourself back at *square one.*

The bad news is that if you are already at the bone-on-bone stage, the damage is done and you will require a joint replacement. If that's the case, after your surgery, make sure you exercise and you will never have hip or knee pain again. However, many people don't exercise after surgery and often end up suffering again. Remember the human body is designed to move, so move. And movement *is* medicine.


## BACK PAIN

Eight out of ten people struggle with back pain at some point in their lives. Back pain is the single leading cause of disability in the world.[19] Given how prevalent it is, you would think we would have some good solutions by now! But most of the time we treat back pain with drugs instead of movement. We block out the pain instead of healing the cause.

According to Dr. Hamilton Hall, author of the award-winning book *The Back Doctor,* 80 percent of back pain is mechanical, not chemical. Drugs cannot fix a mechanical problem; they can only fix a biochemical problem. It is foolhardy to expect drugs to cure a condition caused by unbalanced muscles or congealed fascia. Drugs are designed to block the pain message, not heal the problem.

When muscles are unbalanced, some are weaker than others. The strong ones dominate the weaker ones, pulling the bones out of alignment. The stronger muscles then pull the vertebrae while the weaker muscles don't have the power to resist. The vertebrae becomes off center, leading to a slipped or bulging disc. Ouch! I had two of those. Rebalancing the muscles helps strengthen the weaker muscles to become equal in strength with their counterparts.

Back pain can also be caused by congealed fascia (scar tissue) or damaged discs through compression of the spine. Compression of the spine can be caused from poor posture, slouching, impact sports, lifting heavy weights, repetitive movements at work, construction jobs, manual labor, nursing—lots of things.

According to Dr. Hall, most of the time, correct exercise is the best way to reverse back pain. However, exercise cannot heal back pain that is caused by breaks, accidents, burns, cancers, tumors, or disease.

Arthritis, slipped discs, and bulging discs are three conditions I suffered from in my forties, and I healed them all with these rebalancing stretching and strengthening exercises. It wasn't until I dedicated myself to 30 minutes of daily exercises that I got rid of the constant debilitating spasms. Five years ago, I had an X-ray of my spine, showing that I still had arthritis even though I was totally pain free. These Fast Track stretching exercises have helped me maintain my full spinal mobility with zero pain. I've read many stories in medical journals of people with very twisted spines and severe arthritis being completely pain free. It seems that as long as our joints are mobile and our muscles are well balanced, we can be pain free.

People who do physical labor or work that involves standing a lot—waitresses, hairdressers, cashiers, nurses, construction workers, and teachers—are all prone to stress-related back pain. These workers lift heavy loads and make repetitive move-ments, a recipe for unbalancing and stressing the back.

Another cause of severe back pain is from congealed fascia from sitting too much.

**Prevention and Reversal:** The only way to prevent and reverse unbalanced muscles and congealing fascia is to do a daily routine of rebalancing, stretching, and strength-ening exercises. Due to the fact that the human body is a living machine, it only makes sense that the same healing formula that relieves almost every other type of mechanical pain will also relieve back pain.

Fast Track exercises are designed to permanently rebalance the muscles. Relieving chronic or acute back pain doesn't take long (between a few days to a couple of weeks), but permanent relief from back pain takes a lifetime of maintenance.


## SHOULDER PAIN

Shoulders attach the arm to the torso with two joints, not one. Having two joints makes them able to move in multiple directions, which we like. But that amazing mobility also makes the shoulder prone to injury.

Due to the wonders of modern technology, we no longer need to wash and hang laundry. It's wonderful not to have to scrub the laundry and then hang it on a clothesline, but that means we don't use our shoulder joints as much as we used to. We don't need to grow our own food, which means we don't need to use our arms and shoulders to dig, plant, and harvest. We rarely need to iron our clothes, which means we no longer have that wonderful stroking back and forth of the iron, which kept the connective tissue of our shoulder blades from congealing. We don't need to pick fruit from trees, chop wood for the fireplace, sew our clothes, weave fabric, or knit our sweaters. Many of us don't even need to wash dishes, an activity great for arm and finger dexterity. This inactivity has caused the muscles of the shoulder to weaken and the connective tissue from fascia and ligaments to congeal.

What we do is a great deal of working on computers or texting, both requiring zero shoulder work as we sit slumped, staring at our screens. The tiny movements of our fingers and our rounded back lead to tight shoulder and neck muscles. We spend hours at a time staying quite still as we sit in a rounded slouched back posture. Staying still requires the muscles to support that contracted pose. It's tiring and stressful and quite uncomfortable. After a while (months or years), the surrounding fascia congeals and hardens, creating a rigid cast-like mold to support the exhausted back and shoulder muscles. It becomes difficult to move the arms in their full range of motion, to fully raise the arms above the head or to fully straighten the elbows.

When you don't move, the body freezes. The shoulders are no exception. The less we use the full range of our arms in the shoulders, the weaker they become, until any mobility becomes horrendously painful.

In some extreme cases, the immobility becomes frozen shoulder, which can take up to three years to unfreeze. Movement, correct gentle movement, is the medicine to unlock most shoulder pain.

Prevention: Daily moving of the shoulders, arms, and upper back will keep the muscles balanced and the connective tissue well hydrated so that it's able to continue to slip and slide and move. Nothing is more painful and limiting than hardened fascia or weak, atrophying muscles. The mini-workouts contain easy-to-do arm exercises that you can do as often as you want to reawaken your shoulders, arms, and neck muscles.

Reversal: Take your time as you exercise your shoulders and arms. Move gently and slowly and *never* force. Forcing can cause fragile, dried fascia to tear, creating a new problem. Remember, your shoulder pain didn't happen overnight.

Move in a relaxed, pain-free, gentle mode, visualizing that you are without bones, a rag doll. The floppier and more relaxed you are, the faster the connective tissue will become hydrated and loosened. Each person reacts differently, depending on his or her own individual situation. Feeling frustrated and forcing your body to loosen up could set you back years, so always remember to be patient—you're just getting started.

Whatever you do, don't go out and chop wood or wash all of the walls of your home in the hopes of forcing mobility back into your shoulder. Intense exercises will only exacerbate the problem. Take it slow and easy.

A FULL-BODY STRETCHING, strengthening, and rebalancing program can solve so many conditions. The Fast Track workouts in this book are all designed for full-body stretching, strengthening, and rebalancing. They should serve most of your healing and age-reversing needs.

# PART II

# THE MIRACLE OF MOVEMENT

## THE 30-DAY FAST TRACK WORKOUTS

Are your engines fired up and ready to get on the Fast Track? Good! Over the past twenty years, my team and I have developed and fine-tuned this series of gentle full-body workouts that have the ability to reverse stiffness and "stuck" tissue, reanimate your cells, and strengthen your muscles—and those workouts are now in the palm of your hands.

To get the most out of the Fast Track plan, complete the prep work in the next two chapters. If you're not sure of your fitness level, try the Starter Workout first. If it's too easy, go straight to the Core Workouts. Get ready to start enjoying real, permanent age-reversing results.

# CHAPTER 8

# KNOW YOUR BODY

## *What's Your Aging Story?*

The first step in the Fast Track plan is to understand the science behind why it works so well at turning back the clock. Now that you know the six ways and how they can prevent and reverse the most common signs of aging, you're ready for the next step: identifying your status quo. You've got to know where you are before you can determine where you need to go. Think of it this way: If I wanted to enroll in French language classes at my local university, I'd be tested to determine my current proficiency level so that I could register for a course at the appropriate skill level. Guessing at my level and signing up for a course that was much too advanced (or too easy) would be a waste of everyone's time. Taking the time to establish your current level of health and fitness will help you to figure out the best way to evolve into a younger version of yourself and will give you a baseline from which to track your progress. How do you know how far you've come if you don't know where you started?

At the beginning of all of our teacher-training sessions, participants are asked to fill out a health questionnaire and detail their medical history, indicating where they have experienced pain, injury, or surgery, and providing details. They are also asked to rate their pain levels in the previous two weeks on a scale from 0 to 10, indicating both the average pain level and the highest pain level during that period. We also ask how that pain impacts their daily life.

Then the aspiring teachers are asked, one by one, to share with the class the story of their body: its pains and its problems and the impact of those issues on their ability to move freely, to live fully, and to do what they want to do. I ask participants a lot of questions, seeking details.

Truth be told, I initially get considerable grief from the would-be instructors about this practice. *It takes too much time,* they complain. *It gets boring after a while,* they say. *Isn't it enough to simply fill out the forms as best we can so we can get right into learning how to teach the workouts?* they ask.

*No,* I say. A thousand times no!

Time and again, I've discovered that as we delve deeper into their physical history, participants start to remember past surgeries and accidents they'd forgotten about. Each apprentice instructor remembers and analyzes the life story of his or her body over several weeks. This drilling down into the body's history is enlightening, enabling participants to identify the root causes of the pain they've been carrying for years. Finally they understand why certain parts of their body are stiff and immobile. In this way, the instructors begin to change their own bodies, which is essential to do before working on someone else's.

Over the years, countless clients have filled out similar self-evaluations detailing their health and medical history. It's surprising how most people have gaps in their memory concerning some very serious health and medical conditions they have suffered. We have an amazing ability to block out what we don't want to remember!

For example, when asked about their medical history, people often don't mention an adolescent health crisis or a decades-old injury, even if an unresolved medical problem persists. In some cases, these incidents may have led to trauma and months of hospital stays. They've simply forgotten. But our body carries evidence and memories of every accident, disease, and trauma, whether we remember it or not. It is only by acknowledging that evidence that we can address and resolve it.

When I work privately with clients, I spend a great deal of time with each person analyzing his or her medical, fitness, and often personal history, including habits, jobs, accidents, diseases, divorces, stress points, as well as favorite activities and sports. I watch how they walk, sit, and climb stairs. Everything about their body factors into how they went from having a body that worked for them to having a body that's working against them.

I've included a version of these questionnaires as part of the Fast Track plan because I want you to have the opportunity to get to know your body in a new way. When you have finished answering these very personal questions, you should have a comprehensive picture of what has formed your health from birth to now. You might find out why you are in pain or why you have trouble increasing your flexibility. As you do the 30 days of exercises, you will be able to use this knowledge to understand why some parts of your body are more blocked and stiffer than others.

Fill out the questionnaire before you start the Fast Track workouts. I suggest you use a private diary so that you can make additional notes as you answer these questions. As time goes by, forgotten memories will surface, so keep adding any new personal details to your diary. This ongoing record will help to make your present heath situation clearer. It will also give you a realistic assessment of where you are in your personal aging process and how likely you are to experience breathtaking immediate results or more incremental gains.

Studying your body's history written in black and white will help to shape your expectations. If you've experienced many injuries and are living with an abundance of chronic pain, be patient with the knowledge that healing will happen even if it takes a little time. Remember you can (and should) repeat this 30-day program over and over again. Each time you do, your body will change a little bit more. Gently, over time, this process will nudge your muscles, joints, organs, connective tissue, and bones into better, fitter health. Rome wasn't built in a day, and your body didn't age overnight!

The truth is, the aging process begins the second we are born. Growing from a baby into an adult is an exciting process, but for most of us, it also comes with its share of accidents and injuries. As the years go by, we often forget about these injuries, yet our body remembers. When we don't heal fully from these inevitable bumps in the road, internal scar tissue builds up, growing into blockages in our natural muscle chains and interfering with our ability to move. This impairs our range of motion. Over the years our loss of mobility picks up steam as the original small scar tissue grows into larger wads of scar tissue. When we have reached the point where we've lost too much of our mobility, the stiff feeling makes us act and feel old.

You may be unaware that your body has been faithfully recording its injuries. They remain held in your body as scar tissue blockages until you remove them through gentle movement. The solution is to go back into your physical history, heal your old injuries, and reverse the scar tissue damage. You can go back in time, fix what didn't get properly healed, and move forward with a renewed body.

# FAST TRACK QUESTIONNAIRE

## BIRTH TO AGE TWELVE

These formative years set the stage for your future body's health. During this time, you probably developed eating, sleeping, walking, and exercise (or lack of!) habits that stick with you to this day. Think back and make additional notes in your diary of those habits and any injuries or physical weaknesses that have perhaps gotten worse over time.

1. *Were you a healthy baby?* ____Yes ____No

   If no, describe in detail. _____

2. *Were you an unhealthy child, prone to flus and colds?* ____Yes ____No

   If yes, describe how being sickly affected your life. Did you miss a lot of school? Did you outgrow being sickly? _____

3. *Did you have any illnesses during these years?* ____Yes ____No

   If yes, describe in detail. _____

4. *Did you have any accidents (broken bones, car accidents, burns)?*
   ____Yes ____No

   If yes, describe in detail. _____

5. *Were you in the hospital for any long stays?* ____Yes ____No

   If yes, describe for how long, what it was for, and how it affected your general health going forward into your teenage years. _____

6. *Was there stress in your home?* ____Yes ____No

   If yes, elaborate on what it was and how it affected you (headaches, stomach-aches, depression, etc.). _____

7. *Overall, did you have a happy childhood?* ____Yes ____No

    If not, detail how you feel this affected your health. Try to see if there is a connection to your health today. _____

8. *Were you an active child?* Did you participate in sports, dance, play the piano, or other activities? ____Yes ____No

    If yes, describe what you did and how you felt doing these activities. _____

## AGE THIRTEEN TO NINETEEN

1. *Did you have any broken bones during these years?* ____Yes ____No

    If yes, which ones, how many breaks, and did they heal completely? _____

2. *Were there any complications with the broken bones that are still bothering you?* ____Yes ____No

    If yes, describe in detail. _____

3. *Were you hospitalized for any serious conditions?* ____Yes ____No

    If yes, describe in detail. _____

4. *Did you have any life-threatening illnesses?* ____Yes ____No

    If yes, describe your full recovery period. (Was it painful, did it take years? Are you still treating it? If so, what are the side effects of your condition?) _____

5. *Did you participate in sports?* ____Yes ____No

    If yes, which ones and for how long? _____

6. *Did you get injured playing sports?* ____Yes ____No

    If yes, what was the injury? Were you injured multiple times? _____

7. *Did you dance?* ____Yes ____No

    If yes, did you have injuries dancing? If yes, describe in detail. _____

8. *Are you still affected by those injuries?* ____Yes ____No

    If yes, describe in detail. _____

9. *Did you have feet or hand injuries after playing sports or dancing?*

____Yes ____No

If yes, describe in detail. _____

10. *Do those feet or hand injuries still bother you?* ____Yes ____No

If yes, describe in detail. _____

11. *Did you play the piano or any other musical instrument?* ____Yes ____No

If yes, did you experience any repetitive motion injuries that might still be with you today? Describe in detail. _____

12. *Did you have an eating disorder?* ____Yes ____No

If yes, what affect did it have on your health over time? (Did your muscles atrophy and your bones weaken?) Are the side effects of your eating disorder still with you today? _____

13. *Were you a sedentary teenager?* ____Yes ____No

If yes, has that set you on a permanent sedentary path? _____

14. *Were you overweight?* ____Yes ____No

If yes, how much? Are you still overweight? _____

15. *Were you shy and awkward?* ____Yes ____No

If yes, did this stop you from living an active adolescence? How do you think that affected your body? Did you try to avoid eye contact by rounding your shoulders and dropping your head? Did you try to move as little as possible so people wouldn't notice you? _____

16. *Did you have chronic headaches?* ____Yes ____No

If yes, do you know why? Do you still have regular headaches? _____

17. *Were you under stress at home?* ____Yes ____No

If yes, how did this affect your health and your behavior? Were you always angry? Depressed? If so, have you sought therapy to be able talk out these issues? Do you still carry the anger or depression in your body in the form of tension or stiffness? _____

18. *Were you physically or sexually abused?* ____Yes ____No

    If yes, describe in detail both the physical and emotional trauma. (Remember that this diary is for your eyes only.) Does this abuse affect the tension you carry to this day? Do you have injuries that you haven't fully healed from because you didn't want to revisit traumatic memories? _____

19. *For women: Do/did you have a difficult menstrual cycle?* ____Yes ____No

    If yes, detail how this affected your ability to do sports or schoolwork. Did you suffer from extreme pain? _____

After filling out these first two sections, you will have a better grasp of the basic health you were in at the start of your adult life. Most likely, you were not living in a fresh new body, but one that had already experienced considerable trauma. We tend to forget everything that our body has been through over the decades of our life. The better we know ourselves, the easier it is to be compassionate toward ourselves and gentle with our bodies as we try to reverse the damage of our past.

## ISSUES IN OUR TISSUES

The Fast Track exercises can help to heal old injuries permanently, and the stretching will flush away scar tissue. You can also consciously focus on healing the memory with the physical scar. The use of imagery is a powerful tool to heal the emotional body while you are simultaneously exercising the physical. The best imagery to focus on to heal your emotional body is to love yourself; actually tell your body how much you love it and respect its ability to self-heal. Don't think any self-hating or self-reprimanding thoughts, only loving and respectful ones. Tell your body that you trust it to get better. Make your body feel really loved by you.

## AGE TWENTY TO FORTY-NINE

You may notice that many of these questions relate to stress, tension, injuries, or trauma to your body. Often childhood injuries are not fully resolved or rehabilitated. When a body part is still inflamed, it will carry tension until it is healed; this could last for years. The tension means that we move it less than we do other body parts. This is the breeding ground in which connective tissue congeals and hardens. In time it can literally lock the inflicted joint in place. This imbalance leads to a chain reaction of further imbalance where one part wants to move but its neighbor cannot. So its neighbor becomes locked down.

Connective tissue does not change as rapidly as muscles. Fascia, tendons, and ligaments require slow, patient, gentle movements to loosen stiffness. Muscles strengthen and increase flexibility quite rapidly, but connective tissue is very slow to change and needs to be almost soothed into loosening up.

If you answer yes to many questions about growing stiffer, you can be pretty sure you're experiencing congealing connective tissue. The only way to reverse it is to work slowly, carefully, and in a very relaxed mode. And be patient.

1. *Did you go to college?* ____Yes ____No

   If yes, for how many years? _____

2. *Were you physically active during your schooling years?* ____Yes ____No

   If yes, detail all the various physical activities that you participated in. _____

3. *Were you sedentary during your schooling years?* ____Yes ____No

   If yes, for how many years were you sedentary? Are you still sedentary? Were you semi-sedentary or completely sedentary? Explain what you mean by semi-sedentary and completely sedentary. _____

4. *Did you participate in any sports or fitness programs during these years?*
   ____Yes ____No

   If yes, were you participating at a highly competitive level? _____

5. *Did you have any serious accidents?* ____Yes ____No

   If yes, detail the injuries (broken bones, burns, a concussion). How many accidents? How many broken bones? How long did your recovery take? Were they car accidents? Sports accidents? Construction accidents? _____

6. *Were you physically or sexually abused?* \_\_\_\_Yes \_\_\_\_No

     If yes, describe in detail both the physical and emotional trauma. (Remember that this diary is for your eyes only.) This is the same question as in the earlier section. Please use the same explanation as before. _____

7. *For women: Did you give birth?* \_\_\_\_Yes \_\_\_\_No

     If yes, how many pregnancies? How many births? _____

8. *For women: Did you have complicated births that you never fully rehabilitated from?* \_\_\_\_Yes \_\_\_\_No

     If yes, what are the issues you suffer from today that were not resolved? _____

9. *For women: Did you fully recover your health and the shape of your body after you finished your birthing years?* \_\_\_\_Yes \_\_\_\_No

     If no, in what way did you not recover? _____

10. *Did you spend most of your twenties and thirties sitting behind a desk and taking care of your family, leaving no time to take care of yourself?* \_\_\_\_Yes \_\_\_\_No

     If yes, what body shape or pain changes happened to your body as a result? _____

11. *Did you have a physically challenging job like construction, on-site engineering, or nursing that led to work-related injuries?* \_\_\_\_Yes \_\_\_\_No

     If yes, describe the job and the related injuries and pain resulting from the job. _____

12. *Did you have to change jobs because of injuries related to doing your job?* \_\_\_\_Yes \_\_\_\_No

     If yes, did that lead to emotional stress that may have caused tension that you are still holding in your body? _____

13. *Did you travel a great deal in your job?* \_\_\_\_Yes \_\_\_\_No

     If yes, did that lead to poor eating habits, weight gain, and problems sleeping? _____

14. *Did you gain weight in these two decades?* \_\_\_\_Yes \_\_\_\_No

     If yes, how much? _____

15. *Did you have financial worries that caused a great deal of stress?*

____Yes ____No

If yes, do you still hold some of that stress in your neck, shoulders, and torso? _____

## AGE FIFTY TO SEVENTY-FIVE

Some people consider these decades the best years of their life because they may have become somewhat financially secure and the children have left home. Even if the children are still at home, they probably don't need to be driven around town or have their lunch made. You may finally have some time for yourself. How good is that? However, these are also the decades when the issues of your physical body (that you've been ignoring) start to catch up to you. But never fear: During these next two plus decades, you can easily make enormous improvements to your physical health and reverse many of the negative signs of aging you may be experiencing.

1. *Are you starting to have difficulty getting in and out of a car?* ____Yes ____No

2. *Are you starting to have difficulty getting in and out of the bath?*
____Yes ____No

3. *Are you having trouble reaching into high cupboards?* ____Yes ____No

4. *Are your having difficulty doing basic household chores like vacuuming or washing floors?* ____Yes ____No

5. *Do you feel unstable walking up or down stairs?* ____Yes ____No

6. *Are you unstable when getting out of bed?* ____Yes ____No

7. *Do you feel that you need a cane to maintain your balance when walking?*
____Yes ____No

8. *Did you regularly do yoga?* ____Yes ____No
If yes, for how long? _____

9. *Did you get injured doing it?* _____

10. *What were the injuries?* _____

11. *How long did they last?* _____

12. *Did you fully rehabilitate?* _____

13. *Did you return to yoga?* ____Yes ____No

14. *Did you do Pilates regularly?* ____Yes ____No
    If yes, for how long? _____

15. *Did you get injured doing it?* _____

16. *What were the injuries?* _____

17. *How long did they last?* _____

18. *Did you fully rehabilitate?* _____

19. *Did you return to Pilates?* ____Yes ____No

20. *Did you run regularly?* ____Yes ____No
    If yes, for how long? _____

21. *Did you get injured doing it?* _____

22. *What were the injuries?* _____

23. *How long did they last?* _____

24. *Did you fully rehabilitate?* _____

25. *Did you return to running?* ____Yes ____No

26. *Did you do aerobics regularly?* ____Yes ____No
    If yes, for how long? _____

27. *Did you get injured doing it?* _____

28. *What were the injuries?* _____

29. *How long did they last?* _____

30. *Did you fully rehabilitate?* _____

31. *Did you return to aerobics?* ____Yes ____No

32. *Did you regularly use a treadmill or weight-training equipment?*
____Yes ____No
If yes, for how long? _____

33. *Did you get injured doing it?* _____

34. *What were the injuries?* _____

35. *How long did they last?* _____

36. *Did you fully rehabilitate?* _____

37. *Did you return to the treadmill or weight training?* ____Yes ____No

38. *How old were your instructors?* _____

39. *Did any of your teachers, coaches, or instructors have hip or knee replacements?* ____Yes ____No
If yes, which replacement? _____

40. *Do you garden?* ____Yes ____No
If yes, for how many hours a week? _____

41. *How strenuous is your gardening?* _____

42. *Is your main form of exercise walking?* ____Yes ____No
If yes, for how long do you walk and how rapidly do you walk? _____

43. Are you becoming more sedentary than you were in your thirties?

____Yes ____No

  If yes, how much more? Try to count the hours that you are not sitting. Being in a car is sitting. Eating in a restaurant is sitting (but walking a long way to get there counts as movement). _____

44. Did you have any serious illnesses? ____Yes ____No

  If yes, have you fully recovered? ____Yes ____No

45. Did you have long periods of bed rest? ____Yes ____No

46. Did you require a lot of medication? ____Yes ____No

47. What long-term effect did the medication have on your weight? _____

48. Did your medication make your bones brittle? ____Yes ____No

49. Did you need medication to counter the side effects of other medication?

____Yes ____No

50. Are you still taking medication? ____Yes ____No

51. Have you gone through any personal traumas such as a divorce or a death in the family? ____Yes ____No

  If yes, how did these events affect your physical body? _____

52. Did you carry the stress and sorrow in tension somewhere in your body such as in your neck, shoulders, and back? ____Yes ____No

53. Is the tension still lingering in these places? ____Yes ____No

54. Did the stress and sorrow lead to additional health issues, such as cardiovascular or digestive problems? ____Yes ____No

55. Did the stress and sorrow lead to rapid weight loss or gain? ____Yes ____No

56. Have you begun to have chronic pain in your joints? ____Yes ____No

  If yes, where do you feel the pain? Knees? Hips? Back? Spine? Fingers? Feet? _____

57. *Do your knees hurt when walking up and down stairs?* ____Yes ____No

    If yes, when did this begin? _____

58. *How bad is the pain on a scale of 1 to 10 (with 1 being mild and 10 being severe)?* _____

59. *Have you been diagnosed with arthritis?* ____Yes ____No

    If yes, how serious is the pain on a scale of 1 to 10 (with 1 being mild and 10 being severe)?* _____

60. *Are you still mobile or will you need a joint replacement?* ____Yes ____No

61. *Are you taking pain medication?* ____Yes ____No

62. *Are you taking arthritis medication?* ____Yes ____No

63. *What, if any, are the side effects of the medication?* _____

64. *Have you been diagnosed with osteoporosis?* ____Yes ____No

    If yes, have you been doing regular daily exercise to help reverse this condition? ____Yes ____No

65. *Do your exercises focus on improving your posture?* ____Yes ____No

66. *Are you taking medication to help reverse this condition?* ____Yes ____No

67. *For women: Did you have a difficult menopause?* ____Yes ____No

    If yes, detail all of the ways in which your menopause affected your health, weight, and emotional life. _____

68. *Have you had any problems with drug addiction?* ____Yes ____No

    If yes, what kind of addiction? _____

69. *How much damage did it do to your muscles, bones, and organs?* _____

70. How old were you when you struggled with the addiction? _____

71. How long were you an addict? _____

72. Are you presently an addict? _____

73. Have you had any problems with alcohol addiction? ____Yes ____No

    If yes, are you still an alcoholic? ____Yes ____No

74. How much damage did it do to your muscles, bones, and organs? _____

75. How old were you when you started drinking in excess?

_____

76. How long have you been an alcoholic? _____

77. Have you suffered from fibromyalgia? ____Yes ____No

    If yes, for how long and when did it start? _____

78. Do you have it under control? ____Yes ____No

79. Are you presently on any medication to reduce the pain or discomfort you are experiencing related to fibromyalgia? ____Yes ____No

---

Feel free to add as much detail or as many additional categories as you wish. While you are doing the 30-day program, make it a point to come back to this diary regularly. Often we forget some of the most important events in our life. The better you remember your life history, the easier it will be for you to reverse any lingering damage that these events may have done or are still doing to your physical body.

# CHAPTER 9

# BEFORE YOU BEGIN

## *Set Yourself Up for Success*

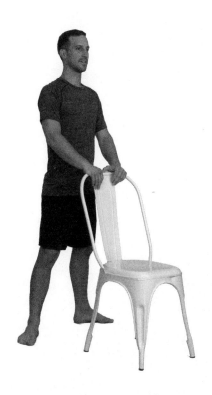

Before you being your workout, either the Starter or the Core, there are a few essentials to gather and keep in mind.

## EQUIPMENT

Here is a list of equipment you'll need for the Fast Track program. Gather these materials together, and the night before you start, place them where you plan to work out.

- A solid chair with a high back that you can hold on to comfortably and that will not fall over.

- A firm, ¾-inch thick mat for floor work.

- Foam yoga brick of approximately 2"x 8"x 12" to be used as sitting risers or head cushions. (For internet purchasing, search for "yoga accessories 2"x 8"x 12" foam yoga brick.")

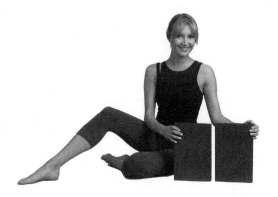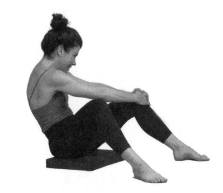

- A firm high-quality stretch or resistance band (or a towel). These are easily purchased on the internet.

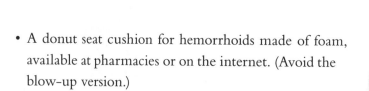

- A donut seat cushion for hemorrhoids made of foam, available at pharmacies or on the internet. (Avoid the blow-up version.)

## PRACTICE GOOD FORM

Maintaining good form is important to achieve the maximum benefit from the workouts. Follow these guidelines and you'll get the hang of it quickly.

### The Correct Way to Hold Your Chair and Stand Beside It

Stand just behind the back of the chair and hold the chair slightly in front of your shoulder, with the elbow slightly bent. Standing beside the chair actually forces you to hold the chair behind the shoulder and drop your weight backward.

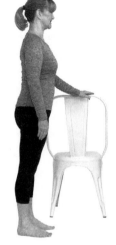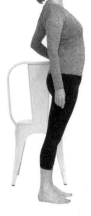

**Correct**          **Incorrect**

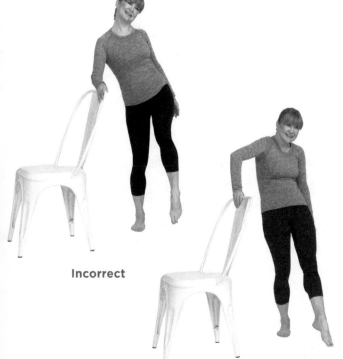

**Incorrect**

**Incorrect**

### The Incorrect Way to Hold Your Chair When Extending a Leg

Do not lean on the chair, bending toward it to support you.

Do not raise your elbow, gripping the chair desperately. This will force you to round your back and lift your leg from the hip instead of from the hamstring.

### The Correct Way to Stand

The correct way to stand is on the soles of your feet. Do not roll your weight onto the outer or inner side of your foot. Doing so weakens one side of the muscles of your leg while overworking the other side. This leads to a chain reaction of joint damage, starting at the ankle and spiraling through the knee, hip, and into the spine. Rolling your feet is often the root cause of ankle, knee, hip, and back pain as well as of arthritis.

Do not roll your feet outward.

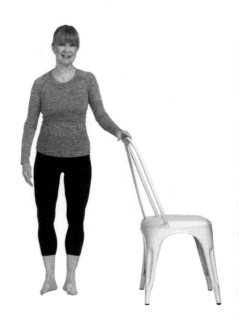

### The Correct Use of the Spine in Forward-Bending Exercises

In everyday life the human body maintains its balance by readjusting the distribution of its own body weight through a *load path*. Whenever we move, we need to make sure the weight of our body flows through a clean load path from the top of our head into the soles of our feet. For example, any time we bend forward, our hips and spine naturally shift backward to off-balance the forward direction; if they don't, we will topple forward.

Unfortunately, if our spine, hips, or knees become stiff, we cannot easily shift our load path. This is one of the reasons why we start experiencing balance issues.

You will notice that in the Fast Track exercises we focus a great deal on the spine, with a primary objective of gaining or maintaining maximum spinal flexibility. The more our individual vertebrae can bend, twist, and turn, the better our balance will be. In this program, we use the position called Neutral C every time we bend forward; it is a position that draws a capital C with the full spine stretching in this forward flexion. The benefit of using Neutral C is that it forces the spine to form a safe load path from head to feet. We use Neutral C a great deal, as it simultaneously protects the spine when we bend forward while also increasing the flexibility of the individual vertebrae.

Whenever a move requires any forward bending whatsoever, learn to go automatically into this position.

You may find it difficult to do at first because your muscles and fascia might have stiffened. In time your body will loosen up. Use a mirror to check that you are positioning yourself correctly.

When you are in Neutral C, you need to round your spine as much as possible, keeping your shoulders, hips, knees, and arch of the foot in a straight plumb line. This is how to create a natural C shape with your spine.

**Correct use of the spine**    **Incorrect use of the spine**

If your bum is sticking out behind you, you are doing the move incorrectly. This causes the muscles of your spine to contract and the weight of your upper body to land on your lower spine. The tension compresses your vertebrae, tightening your back muscles. Tight back muscles are the primary causes of arthritis, bulging discs, slipped discs, and chronic back pain. Work hard on perfecting your Neutral C. It might take a few months.

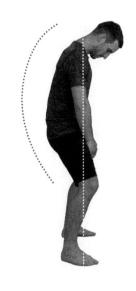
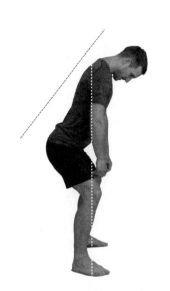

## The Incorrect (Dangerous!) Way to Stretch Your Neck

When stretching your neck, never use your arm to pull the neck into a deeper stretch. This is why: Remember that your arms are capable of lifting incredible weight. Do not underestimate the strength of your arm, which can be used against you when pulling on your own body. The connective tissue of the neck is particularly vulnerable to overstretching, leading to poor posture, chronic neck pain, headaches, weakness, and a dowager's hump. You should never use your arm to pull your head downward in an attempt to stretch the neck muscles.

**Incorrect**

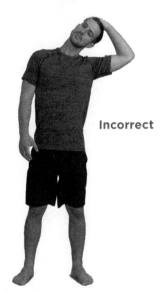

## How to Protect Your Neck When Doing Floor Work

Over time many people have developed permanently rounded upper backs. This program is designed to eventually straighten your rounded back, but in the meantime, you must focus on protecting your neck when lying on the floor. If you have a permanently rounded upper back, it will be impossible to keep your vertebra lengthened as you put your head on the floor. Instead, your head will drop backward as your chin protrudes skyward and your neck vertebra will be dangerously compressed. The easy solution to this dilemma is to place a cushion or riser under your head until you get sufficient support under your head so as to permit your neck vertebrae to straighten out.

**Compressed Vertebrae**                    **Lengthened Vertebrae**

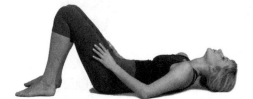     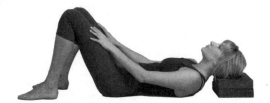

## The Incorrect Way to Do Sit-ups

Sit-ups are designed to strengthen the abdominal and oblique muscles. They are not designed to strengthen or overstretch the neck! In order to strengthen only the "stomach" muscles, you must know where they are in your body.

The rectus abdominis muscles start at your pubic bone and finish around your rib cage. Your obliques are connected to your hips and ribs. None of these are attached to your neck.

**Incorrect**

When doing sit-ups, be very careful not to pull your head forward using the elbows.

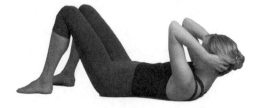

This will cause neck pain, headaches,

and poor posture. It will not in any way help in strengthening the abdominal muscles. It actually interferes with your ability to engage the muscles you are trying to strengthen.

Unfortunately, for decades, coaches and trainers in virtually all schools and sports and fitness disciplines have taught sit-ups using elbows with rapid momentum. Now is the time to start doing safer, smarter, and more effective sit-ups.

## HOW TO GET THE MOST OUT OF THE WORKOUTS

**Do the exercises in the order given and do *all* of the exercises,
even the ones that may feel uncomfortable to do at first**

In developing the Fast Track workouts for this book, I have followed a step-by-step approach. Each of the workouts is designed to systematically unlock your body layer by layer, starting in the outside layers and progressing deeply into your core.

Do all of the exercises in the order that they are written. Don't skip the ones that you might not like or find complicated, as those are the ones that are particularly good for rebooting the brain. And don't change the order of the exercises in the workout.

### Keep the workouts to 30 minutes (add 15 minutes for the floor work)

Do as much of the workout as possible and stop after 30 minutes even if you haven't finished. It is important for developing a habit to know exactly the length of time you will spend exercising. If you decide to add the floor work component, give yourself another 15 minutes to do it.

If you are tired before the 30 minutes is up, stop, rest for a few minutes, and restart. The next day, start from the beginning of the workout, never in the middle or where you ended the day before. Slowly your strength, flexibility, and mobility will increase and you will find these workouts easy to do. Remember, this program is built on gentleness, not force. Take as much time as you need to reboot your body.

### Enjoy your workouts

While doing the exercises, make sure that you enjoy doing them. Find a way to do the moves comfortably. The better you feel while you are doing them, the more you'll look forward to doing them every day. Trust that your body knows what it needs, and when it is ready for you to push yourself, your body will naturally do it.

### Repeat the same workout for at least 10 days

Before starting to exercise, get familiar with the movements by reading the workout sections a few times until you are comfortable flipping the pages over as you flow from one exercise to the next. It will probably take 2 or 3 days to become familiar with each 10-day routine. The better you know the exercises ahead of time, the more you will get out of them.

I suggest you do the same workouts for at least 10 days because it will probably take you 2 or 3 days just to figure out how to do the movements. However, if you feel that you will be better off sticking with the same workout for longer than 10 days, go ahead. It will not interfere with your progress. The most important thing is for you to be comfortable with the movements. You can repeat the same workout as much as you want.

### Slow down to experience fast results

Go at your own speed. I have listed suggested times per exercise, but they are only a guide. There is no rush, and truthfully, the slower, the better. Moving slowly is both more strengthening and safer than moving rapidly, putting you in full control of your body. The slow speed of Essentrics movements protects your body and prevents any possible injury.

### Try a fitness detox

If you are a devoted exerciser and are already committed to doing several other workouts on a weekly basis but find yourself in chronic pain, try doing a fitness detox for these 30 days. If you do multiple workouts every week such as running, weight training, and a Zumba class but are suffering from chronic pain, a 30-day fitness detox might help your body recover from over-exercising. Over-exercising can lead to muscle imbalance, inflammation, and chronic soreness. You will probably find that your body starts to feel better as the imbalances clear up. After the 30-day fitness detox, keep doing your Fast Track Essentrics workouts as you slowly reintroduce your favorite workouts. Carefully monitor which one is the cause of any pain. In this way you can figure out which workout is the one your body doesn't want you to do. Stop hurting yourself and don't do workouts that cause injury.

In most sports, movements are done using the aid of momentum. Weight-training machines, free weights, running, push-ups, and aerobics all use rapid movements. Most of the time when you use speed, you lose the ability to stop your movements in *midair*. For example, once you have thrown your energy into the momentum portion of a weight lift, you'll find it almost impossible to stop in the middle of the momentum flow because of the rapid nature of the movement. In a split second, you go from the start to the finish of a weight lift, a machine pull, a large leap as you are running, or a push-up. If your body is being forced to complete a movement that it may be incapable of doing safely, you may end up with stress injuries to ligaments or tendons or muscle tears.

The slow tempo of the Fast Track exercises keeps you in the driver's seat where you can actually stop any movement at any moment in its flow, in this way preventing potential injury.

### Do not push your limits for quick results

Your age, medical history, emotional history, genetics, personality, and stress level all play a role in determining how long it will take for you to see a change. Some people's bodies change rapidly; others take a long time with little to show for it, and then suddenly their body seems to change overnight. I have learned to never promise how much or how fast any one person's body will change. The only thing I will say is that I have never met *anyone* who doesn't eventually see some positive results when they stick with it.

Now, one important caveat: No matter how intense your desire for immediate results, I cannot emphasize enough the need to work slowly, patiently, and in a relaxed mode. I am aware that these instructions are contrary to what most fitness trainers will say, as they probably encourage you to push yourself to your limit! I encourage you to go *very gently* to your limit. The difference is that one approach can lead to torn ligaments and fascia and the other to rapid healing. Too much enthusiasm often leads to overdoing it—and damage.

Once you begin to exercise gently on a regular basis, changes will definitely take place inside your body. Most of the time they will happen in incremental stages that are somewhat unnoticeable except you will feel better. Then one day you will wake up and your body will feel looser and stronger. You might do the exercises for a full week, experiencing very little in the way of change. Don't let that bother you! Trust in the knowledge that gentle movement increases lubrication and hydration into your fascia, which is the secret to strengthening your muscles.

The human body is designed to be in shape so it will respond as rapidly as it safely can. If you do these exercises in a gentle, slow mode as directed, on a daily basis, you will halt and prevent any *further* negative aging. And if you persist, you will age backwards.

### Take the Mirror Test

Before you start a workout, take this Mirror Test. It will give you an idea of what you need to readjust in your body right away.

Wearing minimal clothing, stand in front of a full-length mirror and have a good look at your body. (Please, when you look at yourself, don't go into self-hate mode. The human body, no matter what shape it is in, is a magnificent living machine. We should all love our bodies and be grateful to have them.)

Are your shoulders level and the same height?

Do you have a slumped stance?

Can you draw an invisible plumb line from the center of your head through your spine, hips, knees, and ankles into the arches of your feet?

Does your torso tilt forward or backward?

Does your chin protrude and your neck curve forward?

Body alignment—how the head, shoulders, spine, hips, knees, and ankles line up and relate to one another—is very important. Poor alignment translates into poor posture and body mechanics. Proper body alignment translates into good posture and less strain on the spine.

Note where you are today in your diary or take a picture of yourself on your cell phone. Repeat the Mirror Test after the 30-day plan. Do you notice any changes?

# CHAPTER 10

# FOR BEGINNER-BEGINNERS

## *The Starter Workout*

I f you are presently in chronic pain, suffer from extreme stiffness, or just feel really out of shape, this Starter Workout is for you. It is designed to safely kick-start your body, preparing it to eventually do the Core Workouts.

It may take you several days to make it through this entire workout from start to finish in 30 minutes. Begin each workout by setting a timer for 30 minutes and stop when time is up, no matter how little of the workout you may have completed. Even a small degree of working out will reap fast results. You'll likely notice a change in your strength and energy even after barely doing anything.

Once you can get through the whole routine, commit to doing it daily for at least 10 days before switching to the more challenging Core Workouts. Take your time to let your body adjust to moving. The objective is to feel completely comfortable and pain free throughout every workout. No pain means lots and lots of gain! Maintain a pain-free mode throughout the duration of your 30 minutes each day.

When you are completely confident in your ability to do all of the exercises with ease and when you find that your body is no longer in pain or immobile, then it is time to step it up and challenge yourself with the next level of exercises in the Core Workouts.

**IMPORTANT NOTE:** In the caption of most exercises you will find the instruction to "Use visualization to stimulate your neurons." Don't skip it! Visualization will help you to execute the movements and is a powerful way to regrow both muscle and brain cells.

# THE STARTER WORKOUT

**REMINDER TO GET THE BEST OUT OF THIS WORKOUT**

Throughout the entirety of this workout, you should be working in a slightly relaxed mode, which means that you release any tension from the muscles, never gripping them, even when the exercise is primarily strengthening (such as sit-ups). A slightly relaxed mode will rapidly strengthen your muscles while liberating your joints and increasing your flexibility. Remember, "Relaxation is the new strengthening." It takes time to master a relaxed mode and do an exrcise workout at the same time, but the results are well worth the effort.

## STANDING EXERCISES

**WARM-UP SEQUENCE**

The warm-up involves five different exercises, each of which should be repeated 16 times. When you finish all five, start again from the beginning. Repeat at least twice. Warming up should last a minimum of 3 minutes. These zero-impact cardiovascular exercises will raise your body temperature by warming up your muscles and releasing tension throughout your full body.

Be sure to maintain a steady deep-breathing pattern throughout your warm-up.

# SIDE-TO-SIDE STEPS WITHOUT ARMS

**Use visualization to stimulate your neurons:** Imagine you are a rag doll, moving with no tension in any of your joints.

**This sequence will get** the blood flowing and your joints relaxed.

**You should be feeling the work in** your legs (especially the inner muscles), knees, thighs, shoulders, and ankles.

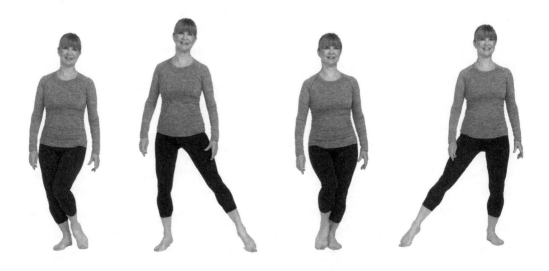

1. Stand with your feet together and your weight on your right leg, with your left heel raised. Keep the pad of your left foot on the floor.

2. Bend both knees.

3. Keep your arms at your sides.

4. Step your left foot to the side as wide as you are capable of doing comfortably, touching the floor with only the pad of your foot. Straighten your knees as you step sideways.

5. Return to the starting position, bending your knees and bringing your feet together before taking the next step. Bringing your feet together will work your inner thigh and hip muscles, and bending and straightening your knees creates a pumping action beneficial to the cardiovascular system.

6. Repeat 16 times before changing sides.

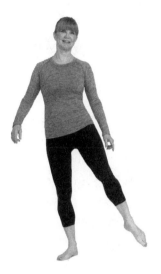

**Incorrect**

# SIDE-TO-SIDE STEPS

**Use visualization to stimulate your neurons:** Imagine you are a rag doll, moving with no tension in any of your joints.

   **This sequence will** get the blood flowing and your joints relaxed.

   **You should be feeling the work** in your legs, knees, thighs, shoulders, and ankles.

1. Stand with your feet together and your weight on your right leg, with your left heel raised. Keep the pad of your left foot on the floor. Bend your elbows and lift them to shoulder height.

2. Bend both knees.

3. Open your arms as you step your left foot to the side as wide as you are capable of doing comfortably, touching the floor with only the pad of your foot. Straighten your knees as you step sideways.

4. Close your arms as you return to the starting position, bending your knees and bringing your feet together before taking the next step.

5. Repeat 16 times before changing sides.

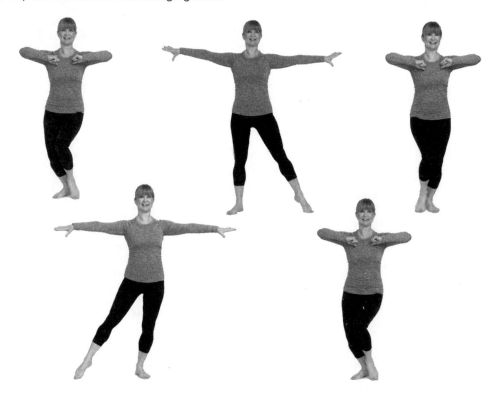

# SWAYING SIDE TO SIDE

**Use visualization to stimulate your neurons:** Imagine swaying side to side in nice warm weather, feeling the wind flow through your fingers as your hands pass through the air gently.

**This sequence will** loosen up the muscles and connective tissue of your spine, shoulders, hips, and knees.

**You should be feeling the work** in your ribs, knees, and shoulders.

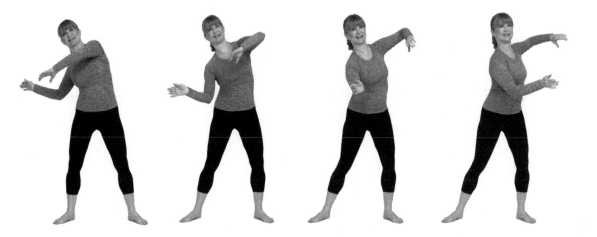

1. Stand with your feet comfortably wider than hip-width distance apart.
2. Bend very slightly sideways.
3. Raise both your arms, making sure that your elbows are bent and your arms are completely relaxed.
4. Imagine that you are sweeping your arms through warm breezy air in a *very* relaxed mode.
5. Let the spine and the full torso sway gently with the movement as you shift your weight from one leg to the other.
6. You will notice that with each sway, your flexibility and ability to bend your spine gets easier and easier.
7. As it gets easier, let yourself bend farther and farther, twisting your body more as you bend sideways and moving your arms as you feel the air.
8. There is no fixed way of moving your arms because they will find what feels most comfortable for them.
9. Sway 16 times from side to side.

# CEILING SWAYS

**Use visualization to stimulate your neurons:** Imagine touching a cloud with your fingertips as you permit your body to sway side to side, shifting your weight from one leg to the other.

**This sequence will** loosen the connective tissue in your spine, shoulders, and rib area. **You should be feeling the work** in your shoulders and ribs.

1. Stand with your feet shoulder-width distance apart.

2. Raise your arms above your head and shift your weight from one leg to the other as you try to touch a cloud with your fingertips. There is no set way to do this; just be sure to keep your fingers, elbows, and shoulders relaxed as you sway side to side, reaching toward the cloud. Feel free to twist and turn as you sway, moving your torso and hips as much as possible.

3. Make sure that you are breathing throughout this exercise.

4. Do a minimum of 16 sways.

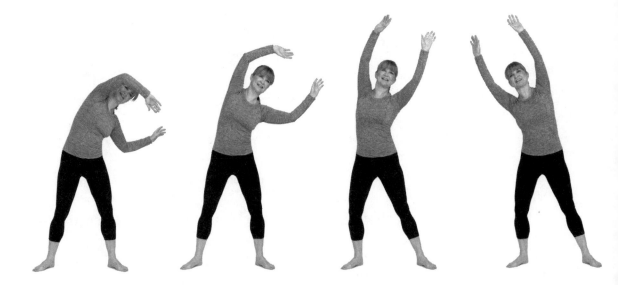

# DIAGONAL SWINGS

**Use visualization to stimulate your neurons:** Imagine your arms swinging like the pendulum of a clock.

**This sequence will** loosen the micro muscles of your spine and the large sheets of connective tissue that surround your entire torso.

**You should be feeling the work** in your spine, upper body, and legs.

1.  Stand on your right leg, with your left leg extended slightly behind you.

2.  Extend your left arm diagonally in front of you, and your right arm diagonally behind you.

3.  Swing your arms diagonally from side to side, dropping them toward the floor as you change sides.

4.  With each movement, you will be shifting the weight from one leg to the other, bending and straightening your legs as you change sides. The bending and straightening of your legs will strengthen your legs and hips as well as pump blood throughout your circulatory system.

5.  Swing diagonally 16 times before switching sides.

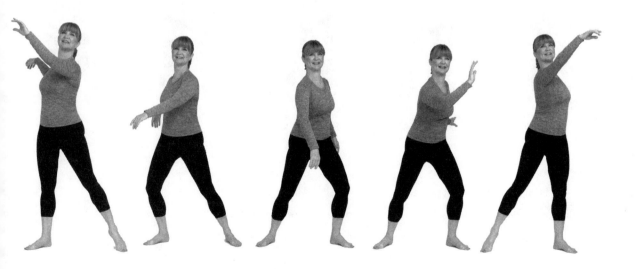

TRADEMARK SEQUENCE

# SHOULDER JOINT ROTATIONS

**Use visualization to stimulate your neurons:** Imagine your shoulder joints as a wheel and that you are going to rotate through all of the spokes of the wheel as you move your shoulders up, down, forward, and back. As you drop your shoulders backward, imagine that you are slipping your shoulder blades into the back pocket of a pair of pants.

**This sequence will** improve your posture, stretch your pectoral muscles, relieve congealed connective tissue in your neck, back, and shoulders, and help reduce a dowager's hump.

**You should be feeling the work** in your shoulders and upper back.

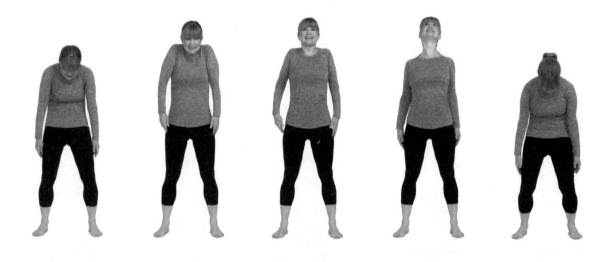

1. Start in Neutral C (page 111).

2. Straighten your back and knees and raise your shoulders as high as possible.

3. Opening your chest as you slowly drop your shoulders backward, imagine putting your shoulder blades into your back pocket.

4. Repeat 4 times very slowly, taking about 30 seconds for each rotation.

**Side View**

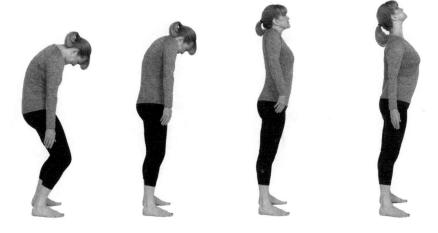

# DIAGONAL PRESSES

**Use visualization to stimulate your neurons:** Imagine pressing against an invisible force, pushing it away from your body with your hand. You can choose how great the force is—for example 10, 20, or 30 pounds of resistance. Make sure that the degree of resistance you choose slows you down while you straighten your elbow and push diagonally at three different heights: shoulder, floor, and ceiling.

**This sequence will** increase the flexibility of your spine and your ribs, improve your ability to breathe, and reduce back pain by rebalancing all of the muscles and connective tissue of your torso.

**You should be feeling the work** in your shoulder blades and joints.

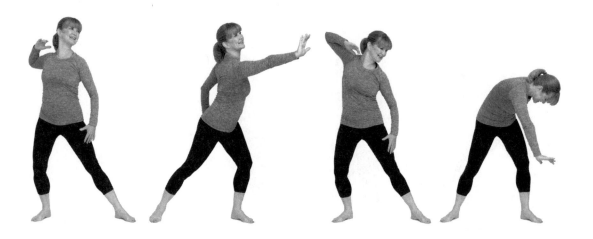

1. Place your feet in a comfortably wide stance.

2. Bend your right leg and your right elbow and lift your right elbow to shoulder height. Relax your left arm by your side and extend your left leg in front of you. This position is used as the transition between diagonal reaches as you alternate sides to center and protect the spine.

3. Shift your weight onto your left leg as you lunge forward, bending your knee as much as possible and pressing against an invisible force at shoulder height with your right arm. The press should take 2 or 3 seconds before your elbow can straighten.

**Note:** It is extremely important to use your knee joints to prevent arthritis and joint replacement surgery. You should never feel pain when you bend your knees, so go as far as you can before pain begins. Pain is a message saying that there is something wrong, which is why it is extremely important never to work in pain. Avoid pain!

4. Shift your weight back onto your right leg and return to the starting position.

5. Repeat 3 presses on the same side, and then change arms and legs, pressing in the other direction 3 times.

6. Repeat this sequence, pressing diagonally toward the floor 3 times on each side before changing arms and legs.

7. Repeat this sequence, pressing toward the ceiling 3 times before changing arms and legs.

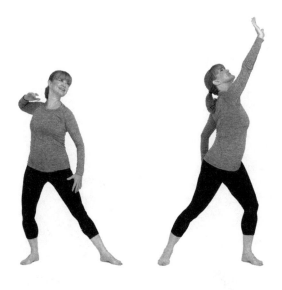

# WASHING CIRCULAR WINDOWS

**Use visualization to stimulate your neurons:** Imagine washing a large circular window that goes right up to the ceiling and down to the floor. Picture yourself holding the wash-cloth in your hands and pressing it against the window as you wash. Visualize this and you will automatically bend your elbows and position your hands properly.

**This sequence will** increase the flexibility and health of the muscles and connective tissue of your spine, arms, and fingers. It will also stretch and strengthen the collagenous protein fibers of the tendons and ligaments in your fingers and wrists. This is extremely important for neck pain, arthritis of the hands, and headaches.

**You should be feeling the work** in your hands, shoulders, and spine.

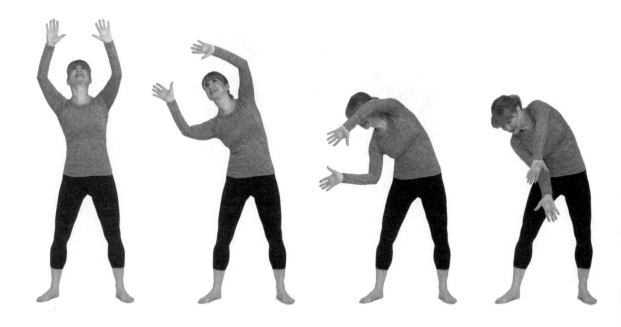

1. Stand with your feet comfortably wider than hip-width distance apart.

2. Relax your knees and bend your arms above your head with your elbows relaxed.

3. Visualize the cloth in your hands, pressing against the window.

4. Move the cloth in a circular motion around the full window from ceiling to floor and back up again on the other side, keeping your elbows bent the entire time. The imaginary cleaning cloth should never leave the window. One rotation should take about 30 seconds from start to finish.

5. Repeat 2 rotations in one direction before shifting and doing 2 rotations in the other direction.

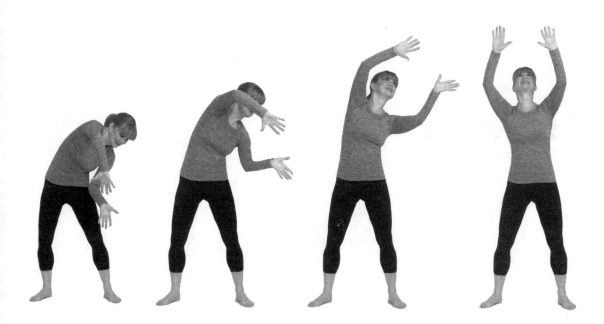

# EMBRACE YOURSELF

**Use visualization to stimulate your neurons:** Imagine giving yourself a wonderful hug, rocking from side to side. This should feel very nurturing, warm, and relaxed.

**This sequence will** improve posture, loosen up tight connective tissue in your shoulders and upper back, relieve back pain, and stretch the entire spine, deep into the latissimus dorsi, which is the largest, strongest muscle group of your spine.

**You should be feeling the work** in your shoulder blades, ribs, and hips.

1. Stand with your feet comfortably wider than hip-width distance apart and with both arms extended out at your sides.

2. Bend your knees, wrap one arm around yourself, trying to touch the opposite shoulder blade. Repeat with the other arm.

3. Stay in this position and slowly shift your weight from side to side as you embrace yourself.

4. Sway from side to side at least 4 times, taking about 4 seconds per sway.

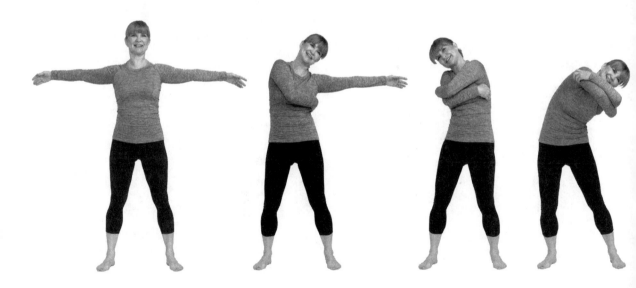

5. Slowly reach toward the ceiling with one arm, relaxing underneath the armpit and pulling the arm more toward the ceiling. As you do so, round your ribs, allowing them to stretch.

6. Raise the opposite arm above your head and reach toward the sky, relaxing your shoulder blades so that there is no tension preventing you from lifting your arm as high as possible.

7. Return both arms to the beginning position and start all over again.

8. One full sequence should take 30 seconds. Repeat at least 3 or 4 times.

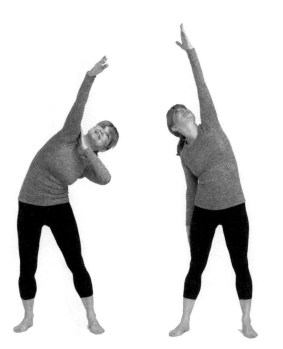

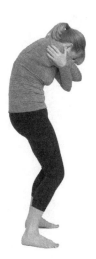

**Side View of Steps 3 and 4**

HANDS AND ARMS

# OPEN-CLOSE STRETCH FOR FINGERS AND HANDS

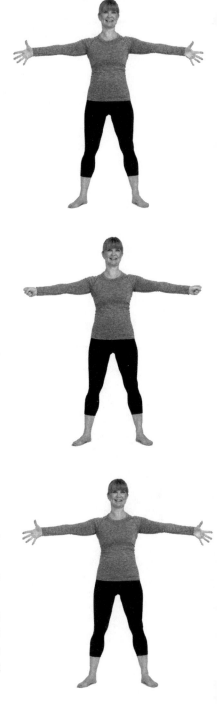

**Use visualization to stimulate your neurons:** Imagine catching a ball and gripping your fist as tightly as possible before rapidly opening the fingers, splaying them as wide as possible.

**This sequence will** stretch and strengthen the ligaments and tendons in your fingers, helping to reduce the pain and immobility of arthritic hands. It is especially good for people who use a computer all day because it relieves the tension that has built up in the connective tissue of your hands that often leads to carpal tunnel syndrome, migraines, and tennis elbow. The results of doing this exercise are really worthwhile, as you will see massive changes in your hand strength and mobility and experience pain relief.

**You should be feeling the work** in your fingers, deltoids, and triceps.

1. Stand with your feet comfortably wider than hip-width distance apart, knees straight, and your arms extended out at your sides. Keep your spine straight and your fingers splayed as wide as possible.

2. Make a fist, pulling the fingers as tightly as you can into a locked fist.

3. Rapidly open your hands, splaying your fingers as wide as possible. Hold for 4 seconds.

4. Force the fingers to open even more. Hold for 4 seconds before closing into a tight fist.

5. Repeat this sequence—hold a fist for 4 seconds, open the hands for 4 seconds, open them farther for 4 seconds—16 to 32 times. Your hands and lower arms will be aching by the time you finish this exercise. Don't worry, you can't hurt yourself doing this exercise!

# FLEX WRISTS

**Use visualization to stimulate your neurons:** Imagine that your wrists are like the opening of a mailbox, able to flap up and down.

**This sequence will** strengthen the muscles of your wrists while aligning the ligaments and tendons of your fingers. It will improve posture and liberate your shoulders.

**You should be feeling the work** in your wrists, deltoids, and triceps.

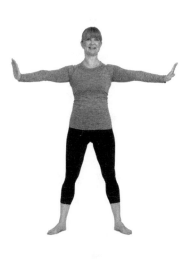

1. Stand with your feet comfortably wider than hip-width distance apart and your arms out at shoulder height. Keep your spine and knees straight.

2. Glue your fingers together and try to straighten them as much as you can.

3. Flex your wrists as much as possible without curling your fingers.

4. Make sure to keep your shoulders down during this exercise, as if you are slipping your shoulder blades into your back pocket. By keeping your shoulders down, you will increase the flexibility and range of motion of your shoulder joint.

5. Keeping your palms straight, flip your hands up and down 16 times, taking 3 seconds between each flip.

6. You will start to feel the discomfort in your underarms and wrists. If the discomfort becomes unbearable, shake out your arms and restart.

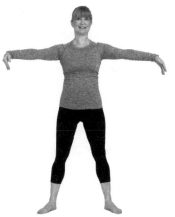

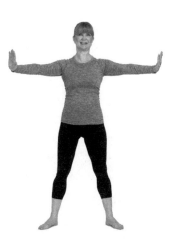

# ROTATE WRISTS

Use visualization to stimulate your neurons: Imagine drawing a circle with your hands as you rotate your wrists.

This sequence will increase the range of motion of your wrists and improve your posture.

You should be feeling the work in your wrists, deltoids, and triceps.

1. Stand with your feet comfortably wider than hip-width distance apart and your arms out at shoulder height. Keep your spine and knees straight.

2. Make a circle with your hands, loosening up the range of motion of your wrist joint. Take about 10 seconds per rotation.

3. Rotate twice forward and twice backward.

4. Make sure to keep your shoulders down during this exercise, as if you are slipping your shoulder blades into your back pocket.

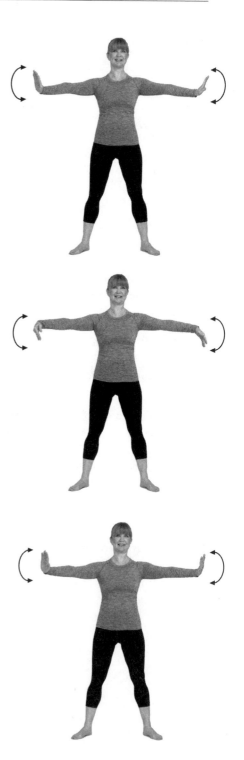

## CHAIR EXERCISES

Remember, the chair is meant to prevent you from losing your balance. Do not grip it tightly or bend forward over it.

### FEET

# FOOT PLIABILITY EXERCISES

**Use visualization to stimulate your neurons:** Picture the skeleton of your foot. You have 28 bones attached at joints. Each has to move separately in order to maintain healthy foot and full-body alignment. As you do these exercises, visualize your joints moving individually and not as an immobile block.

This sequence will increase the health and mobility of the ligaments, tendons, and muscles of your feet. In doing so, it will improve the alignment of your skeleton from your feet through your spine. By liberating your feet and improving mobility, you are starting the process of improving your posture and relieving conditions of arthritis in your feet, knees, and hips. These exercises are very important, as the feet are the foundation of your entire body and they govern your balance. Do not underestimate the value of these simple foot exercises. When your feet are poorly aligned or weak, your body is prone to suffer from joint pain, arthritis, and poor posture and may ultimately need joint replacements.

**You should be feeling the work** in your toes, ankles, shins, and calves.

1. Place both feet in parallel and stand beside your chair, holding it with your right hand. Relax your left arm at your side.

2. Lift your left heel as high as you can, leaving the ball of your foot and the first 3 toes flat on the floor. Make sure the knee and the big toe are aligned. Hold for 3 seconds.

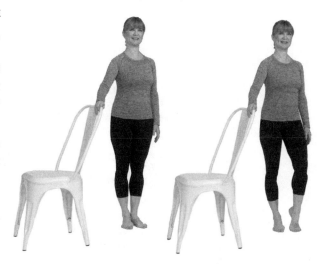

3. Lift your knee so that you can point your toe. Hold for 3 seconds.

4. Keep your knee bent and flex your toes. *Only* your toes—do not flex your ankle.

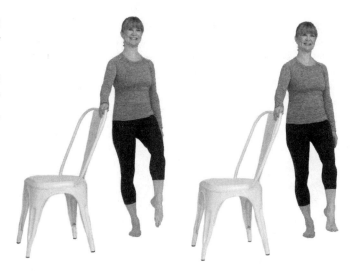

5. Flex your ankle as much as possible. Hold for 3 seconds.

6. Point your toe again. Hold for 3 seconds.

7. Return to the starting position with both feet parallel. Stay for 3 seconds.

8. This whole sequence should take you 18 seconds, from start to finish. Repeat 4 times before changing to the other foot.

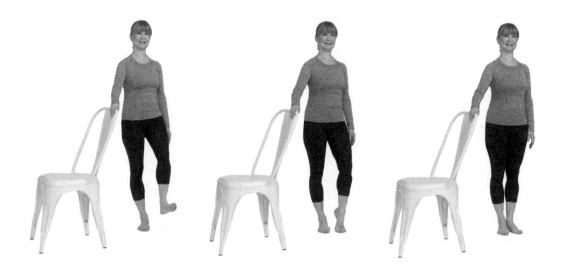

# TOE AND ANKLE ARTICULATION

**Use visualization to stimulate your neurons:** Imagine the joint in each toe moving individually and not as an immobile block.

**This sequence will** improve mobility in your toes and ankle. The ligaments of the toes are connected from the tips of your toes to the top of your skull. When your toes cannot move due to hardened connective tissue, the repercussions of this immobility are felt throughout the body, resulting in stiffness, pain, and potential injuries.

**You should be feeling the work** in your toes, feet, calves, and shins.

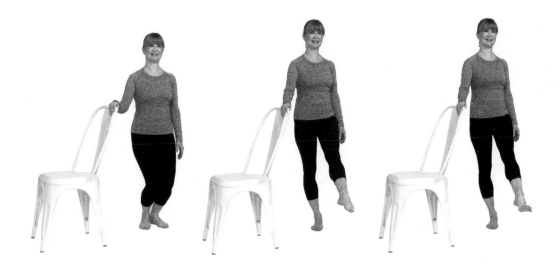

1. Place both feet in parallel and stand beside your chair, holding it with your right hand. Relax your left arm at your side. Bend your knees.

2. Extend your left leg in front, straightening both knees and lifting the leg 2 to 3 inches off of the floor. Hold for 3 seconds.

3. Point your toes. Hold for 3 seconds.

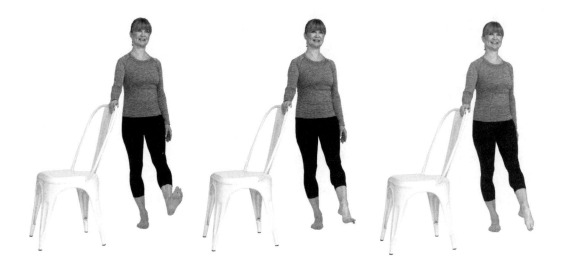

4. Flex your toes. Hold for 3 seconds.

5. Flex your ankle. Hold for 3 seconds.

6. Point your toes. Hold for 3 seconds.

7. Return to the starting position, with knees bent. Hold for 3 seconds.

8. This sequence should take 18 seconds. Repeat 4 times before changing legs.

# ANKLE LIGAMENTS PLIABILITY EXERCISES

**Use visualization to stimulate your neurons:** Imagine your ankle is held in place by hard playdough. You want to loosen up the playdough by making it warmer and keeping it hydrated. If you move too quickly, it will tear. So move nice and slow so that the playdough will loosen up without causing damage to it.

**This sequence will** restore dried ligaments and connective tissue that restrict ankle and toe movement. This is extremely important for regaining the ability to walk and run and live an active life. Immobile feet cause a chain reaction of stiffness and immobility throughout the entire body. When we loosen the feet, the rest of the body becomes more youthful.

**You should be feeling the work** in your Achilles tendon, the sole of your foot, and your heel, calf, and ankle.

1. Hold the back of your chair with both hands. Stand on your bent right leg, while extending a straight left leg behind you. Leave the big toe and second toe flexed on the floor, while the back left heel is lifted off the floor.

2. Very, *very* slowly, try to put your left heel down. Don't force. It doesn't matter if your heel won't touch the floor; it is the increased mobility that counts.

3. Repeat 8 times on the same foot before changing legs.

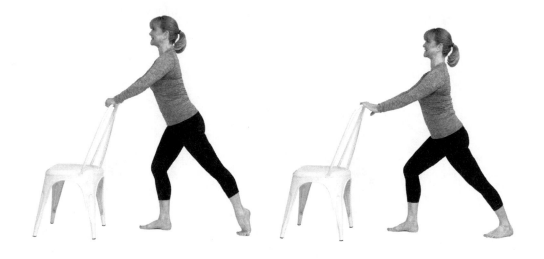

# CALF AND SOLEUS STRETCHES

**Use visualization to stimulate your neurons:** Imagine that somebody is grabbing hold of your calf and squeezing it as tightly as they can for 4 seconds before releasing their grip.

**This sequence will** rebalance your two calf muscles, the soleus and the gastrocnemius. The soleus is a muscle that attaches your foot to your lower leg, while your gastrocnemius attaches your foot to your thighbone. The calf muscle group is what propels us when we walk, climb stairs, and get out of a chair. This muscle group must be equally balanced in order to be able to give us this catapult action that helps us move. If one of these muscles is tight, the other one is also tight. So we have to stretch and strengthen them both in order to get the energy benefits of this phenomenal muscle group. This will also realign the connective tissue in your knee and ankle joints, giving you additional catapult propulsion as you move.

**You should be feeling the work** in your Achilles tendon and calf muscles.

1. Stand facing the back of your chair, holding the chair with both hands, and place one foot 6 inches behind the other.
2. Bend your knees and shift your weight onto the back knee.
3. Begin the exercise by tightening the calf of your back leg as much as possible. Imagine that somebody is squeezing it as tight as they can.
4. Hold the squeeze for 6 seconds, then totally relax your calf, taking 3 seconds to relax it.

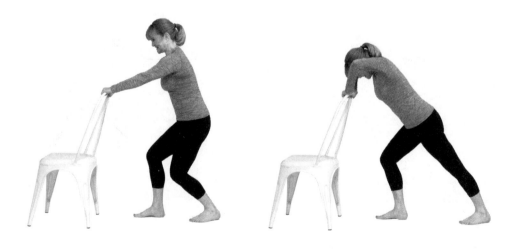

5. Once you have completely relaxed your calf, try to bend your back knee even more. This will stretch your soleus calf muscle. Repeat this 3 times.

6. Straighten your back leg, lift your shoulders and lean forward, pushing your hands downward, trying to press the back of the chair into the floor while digging your back heel into the floor. This will build up a chain of tension between your shoulders, down your back, and into your long gastrocnemius calf muscle. Hold for 6 seconds.

7. Totally relax all of the tension in your back and leg, and try to stretch the calf muscle even more by pushing even deeper into the floor. Repeat 3 times.

8. Change sides and do both stretches on the other leg.

HIPS AND LEGS

# PLIÉS FOR THE QUADS

**Use visualization to stimulate your neurons:** Imagine standing between two panes of glass. As you bend and straighten your knees, the panes of glass will prevent you from bending forward or arching your back, ensuring that you move straight up and down. (If you have very tight hips and cannot turn your feet outward to any degree, you will have to bend forward and backward in order to keep your balance.) Throughout this exercise, pull your whole body upward, trying to separate the joints from one another, starting with the feet and progressing through your legs, knees, torso, and each and every joint in your spine.

This sequence will stretch and strengthen the quadriceps, hips, and ankles. If you have knee pain, arthritis in your knee, or are very stiff and have trouble bending your knees, this exercise is extremely important for you. This is one of the most powerful exercises to reduce knee pain, so do not run away from it. The trick to doing it safely is to bend your knees as much as you can before any pain is triggered. There will be some degree of flexibility even if it is very limited. Over time, as you work in a pain-free mode, your flexibility will increase as your pain decreases. This will improve your posture.

You should be feeling the work in your knees, glutes, spine, quads, ankles, and abdominal muscles.

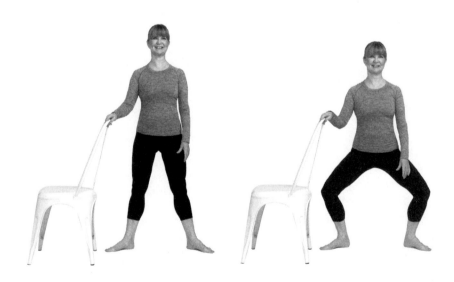

1. Stand beside your chair, holding it with your right hand. Relax your left arm at your side.

2. Place your feet wider than hip-width distance apart, in a comfortable turnout that starts at your hips. Your turnout starts with the rotation of the hips, not with the placement of your feet. Once you find your maximum safe hip turnout, make sure you are standing correctly on the full soles of your feet. Standing on the soles of your feet will automatically protect your knees from twisting.

3. Keep a straight spine and imagine that you are pulling your spine toward the ceiling, lengthening it during this entire exercise. Do not relax this pulling-up effort on your muscles; keep working hard to lengthen them throughout the entire exercise. You will see a huge change in your posture from working in this mode.

4. Bend your knees as deeply as possible, stopping the moment you feel any twinge of pain. Do not let the knees extend beyond your toes. You might have to widen the stance of your feet in order to keep your knees over your toes. It is very good for your inner hip flexibility to keep a wide stance.

5. Take 5 seconds to bend your knees.

6. Remain in that position for an additional 5 seconds and then take 5 seconds to slowly straighten your legs.

7. Repeat this sequence 8 times, or for about 2 minutes.

# PLIÉS FOR THE GLUTES AND GROIN

**Use visualization to stimulate your neurons:** Imagine sitting on a bench, sliding your bum from side to side. Picture the tailbone of your spine and try to move it only to the right, back to center, and then to the left. This will help you to isolate your hips.

**This sequence will** stretch and strengthen your inner thighs and hip joint. It will lubricate any congealed connective tissue, liberating any stiffness that you might feel in your glutes and groin and making walking and sitting easy and comfortable. It will clean out any hardened connective tissue debris that might have collected in the ball and socket of your hip, relieve back pain, and increase the mobility of your spine. All of this will increase your energy!

**You should be feeling the work** in your glutes, hips, spine, and knees.

1.  Stand beside your chair, holding it with your right hand. Place your left hand on your hip.

2.  Place your feet wider than hip-width distance apart, in a comfortable turnout that starts at your hips. Your turnout starts with the rotation of the hips, not with the placement of your feet. Once you find your maximum safe hip turnout, make sure you are standing correctly on the full soles of your feet. Standing on the soles of your feet will automatically protect your knees from twisting.

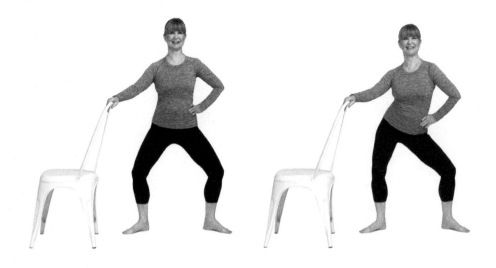

3. Keep a straight spine and imagine that you are pulling your spine toward the ceiling, lengthening it during this entire exercise. Do not relax this pulling-up effort on your muscles; keep working hard to lengthen them throughout the entire exercise. You will see a huge change in your posture from working in this mode.

4. Bend your knees as deeply as possible, stopping the moment you feel any twinge of pain. Do not let the knees extend beyond your toes. You might have to widen the stance of your feet in order to keep your knees over your toes. It is very good for your inner hip flexibility to keep a wide stance.

5. Picture the tailbone of your spine and try to move your tailbone only to the right, back to center, to the left, and again back to center. Move as though you are sliding your bum along a bench.

6. Don't let your upper body move at all; keep your torso straight. Do not bend sideways with the movement. The less you bend your torso, the more flexibility you will gain in your lower spine and hips. It takes concentration to do this.

7. Sway your hips side to side 16 times. Each sway should take 4 seconds.

8. With each sway, try to dig a little deeper in the hips to loosen them up.

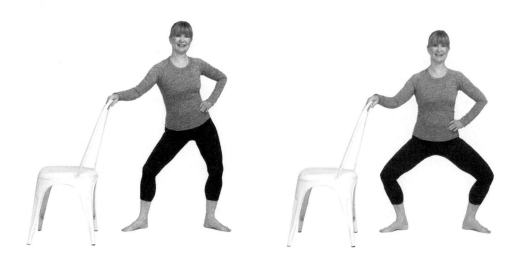

# LONG ADDUCTOR (INNER THIGH) AND SHIN STRETCHES

**Use visualization to stimulate your neurons:** Imagine pulling your bum to the back corner of the room, as you bend slightly forward.

**This sequence will** stretch and strengthen your long adductor muscle (the long muscle inside your leg) and your shin muscles, which are the short muscles in the front of your lower leg. These muscles help to maintain the full mobility of your legs and hips and keep your body well balanced. This sequence will also maintain the mobility of your ankles and hips, making walking and sitting easy to do.

**You should be feeling the work** in the inside of your legs and your shins.

1. Stand beside your chair, holding it with your right hand. Place your left hand on your hip.

2. Bend your right knee and extend your left leg to the side, keeping the knee straight.

3. Bend forward, with a straight back, pulling your bum toward the right back corner of the room. You should feel a pulling on the inside of your left leg.

4. Shift your bum slightly toward the left corner and then back to the right corner.

5. Shift your bum left and right for 8 seconds.

6. Repeat 4 times, for a total of 32 seconds.

7. Flex your left foot as much as possible. Hold for 4 seconds. Return it flat to the floor.

8. Repeat this flex and unflex 4 times.

9. Turn around and repeat this sequence with the other leg.

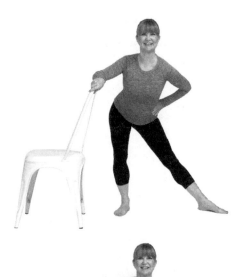

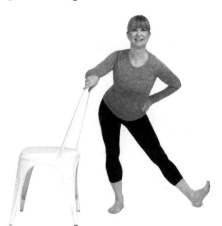

# MUSKETEER'S BOW

**Use visualization to stimulate your neurons:** Imagine that you are a musketeer bowing to the king. Keep your back completely straight when you bend forward. Don't bend too far forward! Pull your bum out behind you, keeping your back absolutely straight, just as a musketeer would when bowing to the king.

**This sequence will** stretch and strengthen your hamstrings, back muscles, and shins. It will loosen the connective tissue group (known as the trousers), reducing stiffness in your hips.

**You should be feeling the work** in your hamstring muscles and shins. You will also feel it tugging around your hips and lower spine.

1. Stand facing the back of your chair, holding it with both hands. Place your right leg straight in front of you and bend your left leg.

2. Flex your right foot and hold it there for 6 seconds as you keep flexing more.

3. Keeping the foot flexed, move your hips gently from right to left, rotating the leg internally and externally within the socket. Take 4 seconds for each rotation, for a total of 16 seconds.

4. Place your right foot flat on the ground and stand up and shake out your whole body.

5. Repeat twice for each leg.

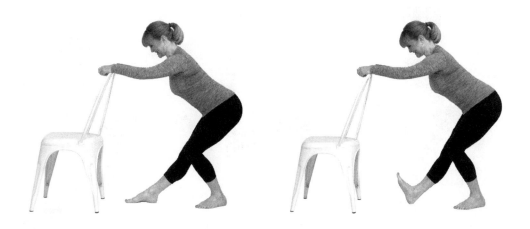

# QUAD STRETCH

**Use visualization to stimulate your neurons:** Imagine your hips as a wheel that you are continuously turning in order to round the lower spine.

   **This sequence will** relieve knee pain by rebalancing the muscles and connective tissue of the quads.

   **You should be feeling the work** in your quads.

1. Stand at the side of your chair, with your right arm holding the chair and your right foot flat on the seat of your chair.
2. Your left leg should be slightly behind you with the heel flat on the ground.
3. Lift your left heel, bend your left knee, and slowly lower it toward the floor. At this point, you will feel the quad being stretched.
4. Think of the hips as a wheel you are rotating until you can't tuck-under your tailbone any further.
5. Go as far toward the floor as you can with no pain. The moment you reach your maximum, return immediately to the starting position. Do not hold the stretch; holding the stretch will have the effect of tightening your muscles.
6. Repeat 3 times before changing legs. This should take you 30 seconds per side.

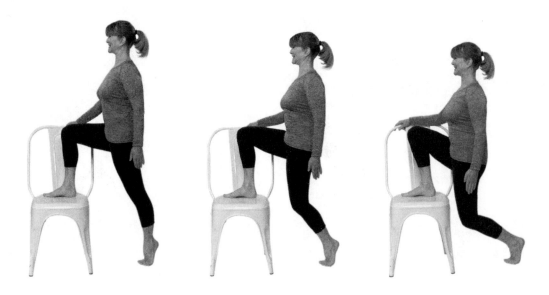

# PSOAS AND QUAD STRETCHES

**Use visualization to stimulate your neurons:** Imagine your hips as a wheel that you are continuously turning in order to round the lower spine.

**This sequence will** relieve back pain by rebalancing the muscles and connective tissue of the hip flexor group, which is composed of your psoas and quads. When these two muscles are tight, they cause compression and damage of the connective tissue of the knees and hips (cartilage) and spine (discs). Imbalanced, this muscle group causes back pain and stiffness. Stretching these muscles will help improve your posture.

**You should be feeling the work** in the front of your hips and quads.

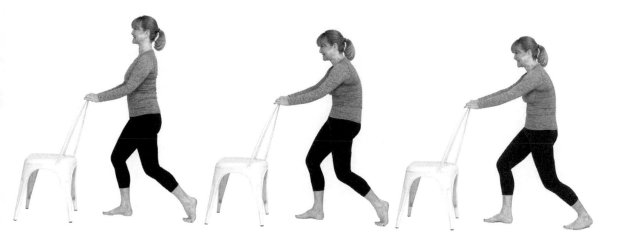

1.  Stand facing the back of the chair, holding it with both hands, with both knees slightly bent and your left leg extended behind your right leg. Your toes should be flexed, with the ball of the foot remaining on the floor. (The ball of the foot is underneath the big toe and the second toe.)

2.  Keep your back pulled up and straight.

3.  Think of your hips as a wheel you are rotating as you tilt your hips until you can't tuck your tailbone any further.

4.  Lock the tailbone in place as you try to straighten the left leg and put your heel flat on the floor. Count to 4 as you do this. If you lock your tailbone tight enough in its tucked-under position, it should be impossible to put your heel flat on the floor. You should feel a stretch in the front of your left hip.

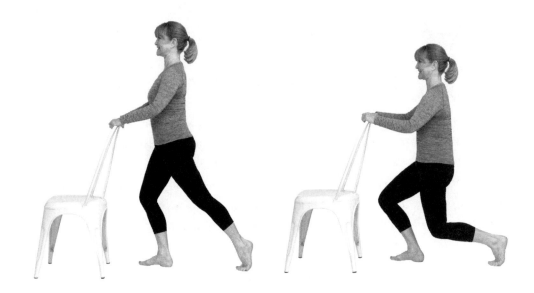

5. Slowly lower your left knee toward the floor. Your thigh (quad) should be at a right angle with the floor, with the knee pointed directly toward the floor. You should feel a stretch in the quads.

6. Lower the left knee toward the floor as much as you can before feeling pain. The moment you reach your maximum quad stretch, return immediately to the starting position. Do not hold or remain in the stretch; holding the stretch will have the opposite effect by tightening your muscles.

7. Repeat the entire sequence 3 times on each leg. This should take you 1 minute per side.

# HAMSTRING STRETCH WITH POINTED AND FLEXED FOOT

**Use visualization to stimulate your neurons:** Imagine reaching as far over your leg as possible to touch the opposite wall.

**This sequence will** stretch your hamstrings and spine.

**You should be feeling the work** in your hamstrings and spine.

> This is an extremely deep stretch. Do not force anything. If you cannot do it with a straight leg as shown in the photos, feel free to bend your knee. This will not change the workout; it will just make it safer for you. Never force a stretch or force your body into positions it does not feel comfortable in.

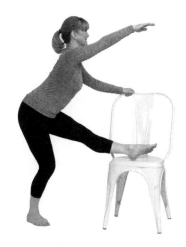

1. Stand facing the side of your chair, holding the back of the chair with your left hand.

2. Place your left foot on the seat of the chair and point your toes. (Bend your knee if it hurts to keep it straight.)

3. Bend your right leg.

4. Raise your right arm and reach over your leg, keeping your spine completely straight. Try to keep your spine as straight as possible. This might be challenging if your back is very tight.

5. Slowly flex your left foot. (You will feel a real pull on your hamstrings as you flex your foot, so be sure to flex slowly so as to not pull any muscles.)

6. Do not let your back or bum round during this phase of the stretch, unless you are incapable of keeping them straight.

7. Take 5 seconds to point and 5 seconds to flex for each foot. Point and flex 8 times before changing legs.

8. Slowly stand up and shake out your body before changing legs.

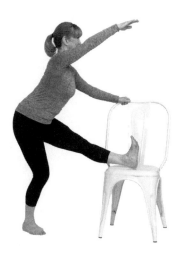

SPINE

# SIDE SPINE STRETCH

**Use visualization to stimulate your neurons:** Imagine pulling each one of your 27 vertebrae apart, using the arm to help pull the spine farther. As you bend sideways, feel each vertebra separating and lifting as you bend sideways to prevent compression of the spine. As you return from the side bend, pull your vertebrae even farther apart so that the return trip upward is even more strengthening than the lowering into the side bend.

This sequence will stretch and strengthen the connective tissue and muscles of your spine and full back. It will improve your posture, relieve back pain, rebalance the body, and lubricate the sheets of fascia that surround your entire torso, giving you a feeling of freedom in your movements, letting you twist and turn and dress yourself with greater ease.

You should be feeling the work in your spine, hips, obliques, and shoulders.

1. Stand beside your chair, holding it with your right hand.
2. Raise your left arm above your head.

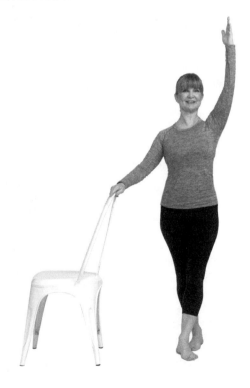

3. Place your left foot directly in front of your right foot, making sure that the soles of your feet are flat on the ground and not rolling in or out at your ankles. You may have to adjust the placement of your feet in order to make sure that they are flat on the ground.

4. Relax your left shoulder to permit the left arm to rise even higher. If you have trouble keeping your legs straight, bend your knees.

5. Slowly reach toward the ceiling, pulling your body upward as you bend toward the chair.

6. Lengthen your body to get a deep stretch through the outside of your torso. Pull the arm out of the socket toward the wall to increase the stretch.

7. Return to the starting position by pulling the arm and the torso upward.

8. Repeat this entire sequence for a total of 3 times.

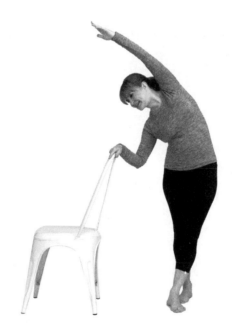

# SPINE STRETCH

**Use visualization to stimulate your neurons:** Imagine that your spine is a stairway and you are going to walk up and down each vertebra one at a time.

**This sequence will** stretch the spine, relieve back pain, and improve your posture.

**You should be feeling the work** in your hamstrings, spine, and shoulders.

> This is a wonderful stretch for your spine. Do not worry if you cannot bend and straighten your spine as pictured. It could be due to tight muscles or congealed connective tissue. In time, your spine will release the tension and you will able to stand straighter.

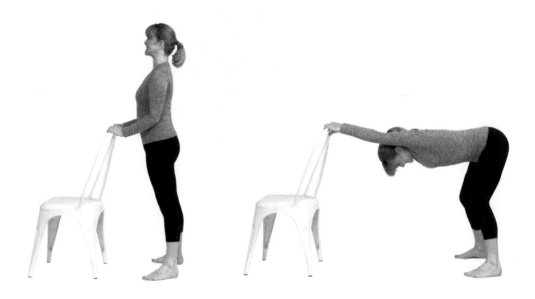

1. Stand facing the back of your chair. Place your feet apart and hold the back of the chair with both hands.

2. Keeping your hands on the back of the chair, walk backward as you bend forward.

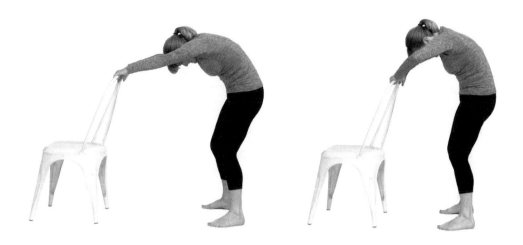

3. Finish with both knees bent, feet more than hip-width distance apart and arms and spine horizontal with the floor. If you have a very tight spine, you may not be able to straighten your spine to make it horizontal with the floor. Not to worry, do the best you can. In time this exercise will help you straighten your spine.

4. Very, *very* slowly, tuck your tailbone under and roll up your spine as you take tiny steps forward.

5. This little walk forward should take about 15 seconds. You want to feel every vertebra as you move toward the chair.

6. This sequence will end in the same position that it began. From start to finish, it should take 30 seconds.

# DIAGONAL SPINE STRETCH

**Use visualization to stimulate your neurons:** Imagine getting ready in the morning and putting your hands on the bathroom sink as you bend forward to give yourself a natural, relaxing massage-type movement. We all know it feels great first thing in the morning to stretch out our backs. Do this stretch with that in mind!

**This sequence will** work the full sheets of connective tissue from your shoulders to your knees, lubricating and liberating any congealed fascia. It should feel really, really good. If it doesn't feel good, adjust!

**You should be feeling the work** through your entire back and into your hips.

1. Hold the back of the chair with both hands, standing far enough away from the chair so that you can round your back completely and extend your elbows. Your feet should be wider than hip-width distance apart.

2. Round your back, bend your knees, and tuck your tailbone under.

3. Shift your weight onto your right leg, bending the right leg more than the left leg so that one side of the torso gets more stretched. Wiggle around in that position, getting a self-massage, for 4 to 5 seconds.

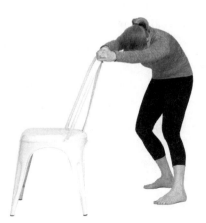

4. Without moving the position of your feet, shift your weight onto the left leg, bending it more than the right. Repeat wiggling around for 4 to 5 seconds so that you give yourself a self-massage of the muscles on this side of the torso.

5. Repeat at least 3 times, side to side. This should be a feel-good exercise.

6. The complete sequences should take about 30 to 45 seconds. Take your time and enjoy this stretch.

# NECK AND CHEST STRETCH

**Use visualization to stimulate your neurons:** Imagine stretching your head away from your neck, pulling each vertebra apart as you stretch the spine upward.

**This sequence will** liberate tight necks, relieve neck and upper back pain, and reduce headaches.

**You should be feeling the work** in your neck and shoulder muscles.

---

- It is extremely important that you do not let your cervical spine (the neck region of the spine) release the upward pull or permit your skull to drop backward. This could compress the vertebra and weaken the neck portion of your spine.

- If you find it difficult to tilt your face upward, it could be because your neck and shoulder muscles are tight or the surrounding connective tissue is somewhat congealed. Do not try to force higher than you are comfortably capable of. Many people can barely move. That's okay. Gentle correct movement will safely liberate congealed connective tissue and tight muscles a little bit at a time. The changes may be so minuscule that you won't notice them at first, so don't worry if at first nothing seems to be loosening.

---

1. Stand facing the back of your chair, holding the chair with both hands. Feet should be hip-width distance apart. Look straight in front of you.
2. Slowly tilt your face toward the ceiling, lifting it upward.
3. As you tilt your head to face the ceiling, simultaneously pull your spine upward.

4. Tilt your head back to the starting position, but continue trying to lengthen the spine. Do not release the pull upward on your vertebrae throughout this exercise.

5. Repeat 4 times. Each head tilt should take about 15 seconds from start to finish.

6. Finish by shaking your head and shoulders to relax.

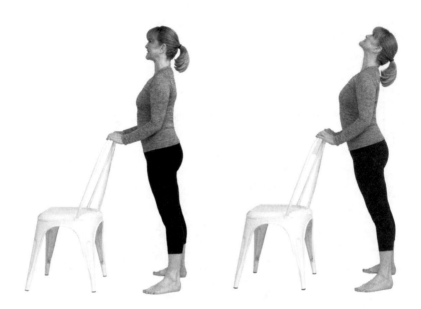

SEATED STRETCHES

# SEATED SPINE STRETCH WITH DEEP BREATHING

**Use visualization to stimulate your neurons:** Imagine that you are sitting on your chair and somebody behind you hails you and you turn your head and torso to look back at them. Don't move quickly!

**This sequence will** increase the range of motion of your spine, liberating the tiny muscles that tend to atrophy and block rotation. It will lubricate and liberate the sheets of fascia that surround your torso, making spine mobility comfortable and easy. We use deep breathing in this sequence in order to safely and comfortably increase your spinal flexibility.

**You should be feeling the work** in your hips, spine, rhomboids, and shoulders.

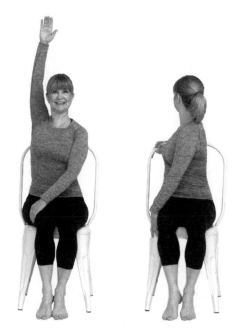

1. Sit on the chair with your legs together, feet flat on the ground.
2. Hold your right leg with your left hand and reach your right arm to the ceiling, counting to 4.
3. Start the breathing sequence here.
4. Sitting facing the front, inhale, counting to 4.

5. As you exhale, count to 4 while you rotate toward the back of the room, pulling the spine toward the ceiling. Grasp the seat, arms, or back of the chair to assist your rotation.

6. You should now be looking at the back of the room and twisting your spine.

7. Inhale for 4 counts as you hold the back of the chair.

8. As you exhale, count to 4 while you use the back of the chair as a lever, trying to twist the spine even further.

9. Inhale for 4 counts as you lift your right arm above your head and return to the front.

10. Repeat the entire sequence 3 times on each side.

# SEATED HIPS AND GLUTES STRETCH

**Use visualization to stimulate your neurons:** Imagine using the massage-like motion you would use to knead dough on your hip muscles. This massage-like movement will assist in loosening congealed fascia and tight muscles.

**This sequence will** work into the deep connective tissue of the hips (the ligaments, cartilage, and fascia).

**You should be feeling the work** in your hips.

1. Sit on your chair and try to put the ankle of your right leg onto your left thigh. If you have trouble doing this, just lift your knee as close as you can toward your chest.

2. Take your right hand and gently push down on the thigh, just above the knee joint. Push very gently. This will stretch your hip muscles (glutes).

3. Keep pushing for about 5 seconds.

4. Take your right knee and pull it toward your chest.

5. With your left hand, hold the shinbone of your right leg, trying to pull it toward your stomach.

6. As you are doing this, shift your hips on the chair several times, as though you are kneading dough.

7. Do this stretch for at least 5 seconds.

8. Repeat this complete sequence 3 times for a total of 30 seconds on each leg.

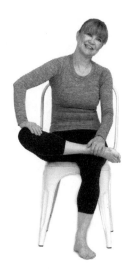

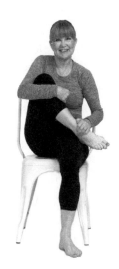

# SEATED HAMSTRING STRETCH

Use visualization to stimulate your neurons: Imagine that every time you slowly straighten and bend the long wide elastic-band type muscles of your hamstrings, a massive inflow of fluid rushes into the muscles hydrating them, increasing both their strength and flexibility.

This sequence will stretch your hamstrings and glutes, improving your posture, liberating any tension in your knees and hips, and relieving pain. This exercise is extremely beneficial for people who suffer from back pain. When you increase the flexibility of your hamstrings, you will have greater ease and comfort walking, climbing stairs, and generally moving around. Flexible hamstrings also make it easier for you to get on and off a chair and in and out of a car. As your final exercise of the Starter Workout, it should leave you feeling energized and lighter.

You should be feeling the work in your hamstrings and hips.

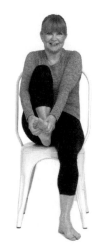

1. Sit on your chair. Lifting your right leg, bend the knee as you pull it toward your chest. Hold the sole of your foot with both hands, your spine rounded. If you cannot hold your foot, wrap a towel or a stretch band around your foot in order to lift it up.

2. Holding the foot or stretch band, try to slowly straighten the right knee. Take 5 seconds.

3. You will feel this stretch in your hamstring muscle (the muscle under your leg) and your hips. Don't force it! The moment you feel a stretch, that's good enough.

4. Bend your knee, returning to the starting position. Wiggle your hips to take any tension out of your muscles. Rest there for 5 seconds.

5. Repeat 4 times for each leg.

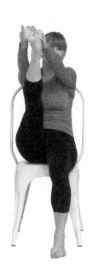

# CHAPTER 11

# FOR ACTIVE ADULTS

## *The 30-Day Fast Track Core Workouts*

The Core Workouts offer powerful age-reversing benefits: energy, vitality, and mobility. These workouts will give you a bounce in your step and a youthful zing to all your movements. They are absolutely for everyone!

The Core Workouts are comprised of three 10-day workouts. Each workout has two distinct parts.

Part One in each workout consists of Standing and Chair Exercises. Part One is essential and suitable for all levels of fitness. It includes exercises done standing and using a chair to stretch and strengthen your muscles; hydrate and liberate your connective tissue; and align your joints. It is important to recognize that exercising your connective tissue requires a deliberately slow pace. This slow speed gives the layers of fascia sufficient time to unglue and rebuild the essential slipping and sliding action between them. Rapid movements such as aerobics, running, or weight training are useless in loosening congealed fascia or repairing damaged connective tissue. This is why we are moving slowly. Only by rebuilding and rehydrating all your connective tissue will you be able to regain lost mobility to enjoy age-reversing results.

Part One of each of these workouts should take you about 30 minutes.

If you feel that after doing Part One you have worked sufficiently for your needs, stop there. Be assured, Part One gives you the full benefits of healing and age-reversing. In this program we encourage people to never push beyond their comfort level, as over the weeks you will develop increased strength and energy. This gentle approach achieves faster results.

Part Two of each workout involves Floor Exercises. Part Two is for people who self-identify as intermediate or advanced and are strong and energetic enough to push a little harder. These exercises are aimed at toning, stretching, and strengthening. If you are struggling with Part One, hold off on Part Two until you feel strong enough. The key to aging backwards is to fully understand that the archaic mantra of "no pain, no gain" is unhealthy and self-defeating and should be relegated to the dustbin of history! Only when you find Part One easy should you add the floor work exercises in Part Two.

Go at your own pace. Don't push yourself to do both parts until you are *completely* comfortable finishing Part One.

The most important advice is to never skip the standing and chair exercises, believing that the toning exercises are the ones that will give you a sexy, toned body—it doesn't work that way! The dramatic results from the toning exercises require the hydrating, liberating, and strengthening in Part One to work.

---

**IMPORTANT NOTE:** In the captions of most exercises you will find the instruction to "Use visualization to stimulate your neurons." Don't skip these directions! Visualization will help you to effectively and rapidly execute the movements, as well as being a proven method to regrow both muscle and brain cells.

A reminder to get the best out of these workouts by working in a slightly relaxed mode. Remember, "Relaxation is the new strengthening."

# WORKOUT 1: DAYS 1–10

## PART ONE OF WORKOUT 1: Standing and Chair Exercises

## PART TWO OF WORKOUT 1: Floor Exercises (optional)

### PART ONE OF WORKOUT 1: **Standing and Chair Exercises**

## STANDING EXERCISES

**WARM-UP SEQUENCE**

The warm-up involves five different exercises, each of which should be repeated 16 times. When you finish all five, start again from the beginning. Repeat at least twice. Warming up should last a minimum of 3 minutes. These zero-impact cardiovascular exercises will raise your body temperature by warming up your muscles and releasing tension throughout your full body.

Be sure to maintain a steady deep-breathing pattern throughout your warm-up.

# SWAYING SIDE TO SIDE

**Use visualization to stimulate your neurons:** Imagine swaying side to side in nice warm weather, feeling the wind flow through your fingers as your hands pass through the air gently.

**This sequence will** loosen up the muscles and connective tissue of your spine, shoulders, hips, and knees.

**You should be feeling the work** in your ribs, knees, and shoulders.

1. Stand with your feet comfortably wider than hip-width distance apart.
2. Bend very slightly sideways.
3. Raise both your arms, making sure that your elbows are bent and your arms are completely relaxed.
4. Imagine that you are sweeping your arms through warm breezy air in a *very* relaxed mode.
5. Let the spine and the full torso sway gently with the movement as you shift your weight from one leg to the other.
6. You will notice that with each sway, your flexibility and ability to bend your spine will improve.

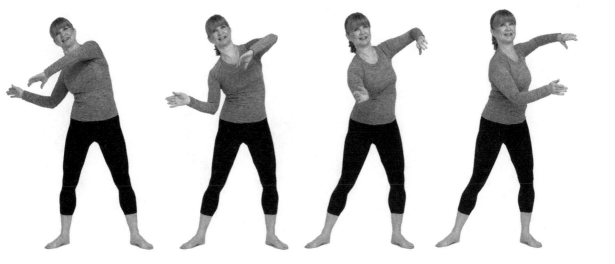

7. As it gets easier, let yourself bend farther and farther, twisting your body more as you bend sideways and moving your arms as you feel the air.

8. There is no fixed way of moving your arms because they will find what feels most comfortable for them.

9. Sway 16 times from side to side.

# DIAGONAL SWINGS

**Use visualization to stimulate your neurons:** Imagine your arms swinging like the pendulum of clock.

**This sequence will** loosen the micro muscles of your spine and the large sheets of connective tissue that surround your entire torso.

**You should be feeling the work** in your spine, upper body, and legs.

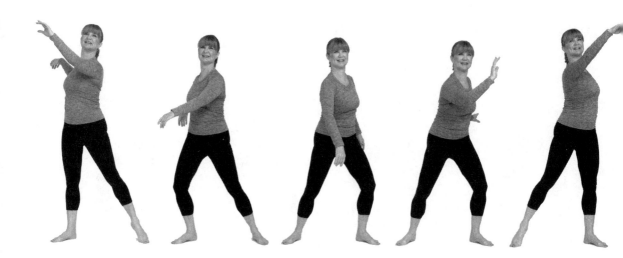

1. Stand on your right leg with your left leg extended slightly behind you. Raise your left arm diagonally in front of you and your right arm diagonally behind you as you twist on your spine.

2. In a very relaxed mode, start shifting your weight onto your left leg, bending both knees and lowering your arms toward your thighs.

3. Slowly rotate your spine in the other direction as you raise your right arm diagonally in front of you and your left arm behind you.

4. Repeat shifting from right to left 16 times, rotating your spine as you lift your arms diagonally.

5. Move slowly and remain in a relaxed mode throughout.

# SIDE-TO-SIDE STEPS WITH THREE ARM VARIATIONS

**Use visualization to stimulate your neurons:** Imagine you are a rag doll, moving with no tension in any of your joints.

**This sequence will** increase your ability to twist your spine by warming up all of the vertebrae and the surrounding muscles and connective tissue.

**You should be feeling the work** in your core as you twist and in your thighs and glutes as you bend and straighten your legs.

**Variation 1**

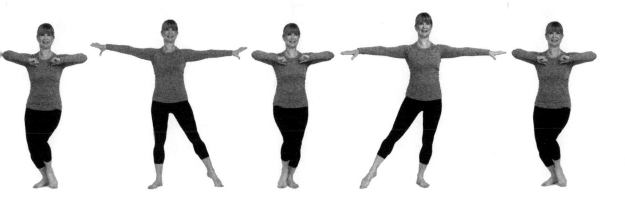

1. Stand with your feet together and your weight on your right leg, with your left heel raised. Keep the pad of your left foot on the floor.

2. Bend both knees.

3. Open your arms as you step your left foot to the side as wide as you are capable of doing comfortably, touching the floor with only the pad of your foot. Straighten your knees as you step sideways.

4. Close your arms as you return to the starting position, bending your knees and bringing your feet together before taking the next step.

5. Repeat 16 times before changing sides.

**Variation 2**

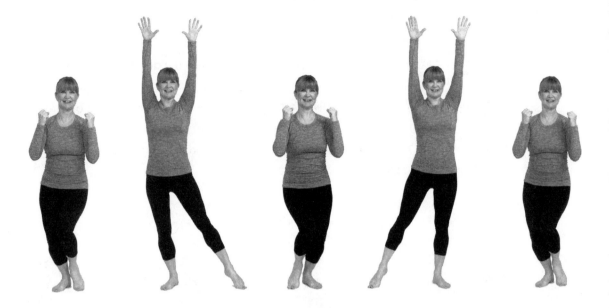

1. Doing the same legwork as in the previous sequence, start with your left leg slightly bent and your arms bent at the elbows so that your thumbs come up to your shoulders.

2. As you extend your left leg out sideways, reach both arms up in the air.

3. Bring your arms back down, bend at the elbows, and shift your weight so that your right knee is slightly bent.

4. Extend your right leg out and reach both arms up in the air.

5. Repeat this sequence 16 times.

**Variation 3**

1. Doing the same legwork as in the previous sequence, start with your left leg slightly bent and your arms bent at the elbows so that your thumbs come up to your shoulders.

2. Extend your left leg out sideways and straighten your arms down to touch your thighs.

3. Bring your left leg back to center and bend your right knee, bending your arms at the same time.

4. Extend your right leg out sideways and straighten your arms down to your thighs.

5. Repeat this sequence 16 times.

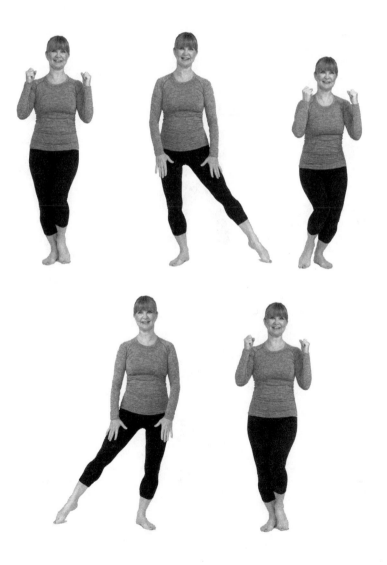

TRADEMARK SEQUENCE

# SPINAL ROLL INTO AN OPEN CHEST SWAN

**Use visualization to stimulate your neurons:** Imagine rolling up one vertebra at a time.

This sequence will stretch and strengthen the entire musculature and connective tissue of your torso. It will relieve back and shoulder pain while improving posture.

You should be feeling the work in the sheets of connective tissue in your back and chest (latissimus dorsi, erector spinae, pectorals, shoulder girdle, and gluteus maximus). Try to actually feel each individual vertebra as you stack them one on top of the other.

**Front View**

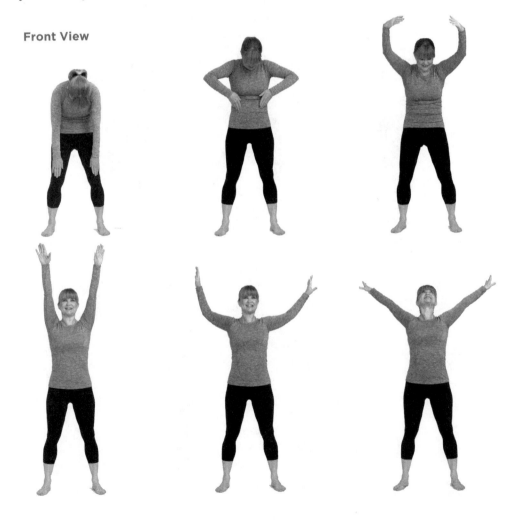

1. Stand with your legs slightly wider than hip-width distance apart and knees bent.

2. Find the most comfortable placement for your feet.

3. Try to round your spine by tucking your tailbone under and pushing the middle of your spine back. Raise your shoulders, pulling them in front of you. (Note: This is not a forward bend, this is a spine stretch.)

4. Slowly straighten your spine by rolling up one vertebra at a time. This should take a minimum of 10 seconds.

5. As you roll up, let your hands touch the front of your body, moving up to your shoulders and then raising your arms above your head.

6. Reach your arms as high as you can toward the ceiling. Make sure to keep your weight slightly forward to prevent sinking into your lower spine.

7. Relax your shoulders, relax your torso, and stretch the arms toward the ceiling. The more relaxed you are, the higher you will be able to reach. This ceiling reach should last between 7 and 10 seconds.

8. Carefully bend your elbows, pulling them toward the back of the room. Imagine that you are dropping your shoulder blades into your back pocket. This should take 4 to 5 seconds.

9. Slowly straighten the elbows, reaching toward the back of the room as though you are stroking the air with the wings of a magnificent swan.

10. Lower your arms and repeat the full sequence 4 times.

**Side View**

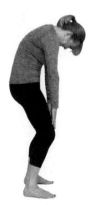
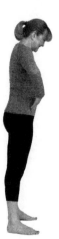
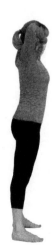

# EMBRACE A BEACH BALL

**Use visualization to stimulate your neurons:** Imagine pulling a giant beach ball close to your body as you follow its circumference with both hands. Imagine that the beach ball is almost weightless so that you don't have to tense up your muscles. Keep both the weight and circumference of the ball in your mind the entire time you do this sequence.

**This sequence will** work through every vertebra in your spine while liberating the connective tissue and muscles from your heels to your skull. It will improve your posture.

**You should be feeling the work** throughout your spine and between your shoulder blades as well as in your glutes and thighs.

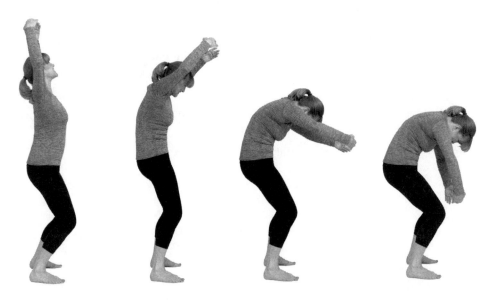

1. Stand with your legs slightly wider than hip-width distance apart, with your feet settled comfortably on the floor. Some people are more comfortable with their toes turned slightly in and others prefer their toes to be slightly turned out. You choose the position that works best for you.

2. Bend your knees.

3. Raise your arms above your head as if you are holding a beach ball. Your arms should be bent so that they can circle around the ball. Open your fingers as wide as possible to prevent the beach ball from slipping out of your embrace. This stretches the ligaments and tendons of your fingers, releasing sheets of connective tissue from your arms to your neck and spine.

4. Tuck your tailbone under and round your entire spine. Keep the front of your torso, from chest to stomach, glued to the ball. Visualizing the ball will keep your spine in a rounded position.

5. Slowly roll up on your spine, one vertebra at a time. Try not to bend forward too much as you hold the beach ball with your arms.

6. When your hands reach your shoulders, let the beach ball go while you straighten your arms above your head, your spine, and your legs.

7. Slowly straighten the elbows, reaching toward the back of the room as though you are stroking the air with the wings of a magnificent swan.

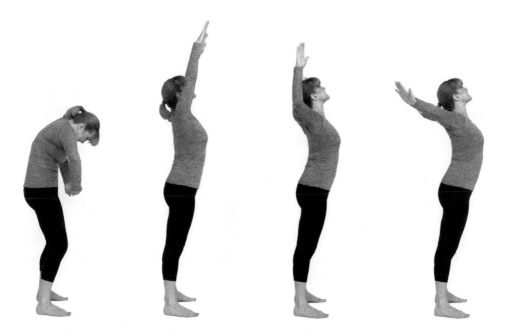

8. Raise your arms above your head to return to the starting position.

9. It should take you 30 seconds to do this entire sequence.

10. Repeat this complete sequence 4 times.

# HALF ROTATION OF THE TORSO

**Use visualization to stimulate your neurons:** Imagine using the full length of your arm to draw a large semicircle over your head from one shoulder to the other, and then extending the circle in front of you, again from one shoulder to the other.

This sequence will stretch, strengthen, and tone your waist, arms, and back. It's good for losing inches, regaining lost height, and relieving back pain.

You should be feeling the work in your entire torso.

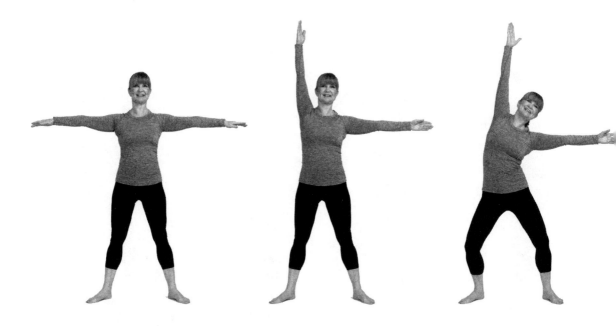

1. Start with your legs much wider than hip-width distance apart (approximately three times the length of your foot). If this causes pain, reduce the spread so you are pain free.

2. Your feet should be comfortably turned out on the floor. The degree of safe turnout varies from person to person. With the correct foot placement, you shouldn't feel any stress in your hips, knees, or feet. Adjust your feet accordingly and choose the degree of turnout that works best for you.

3. Your knees are straight.

4. Extend both of your arms to shoulder height with straight elbows.

5. Raise your right arm above your head. Hold your left arm at shoulder height.

6. Bend your knees and reach to the ceiling while bending your torso to the left.

7. Shift your weight onto your bent left leg, straightening your right leg.

8. Bend much farther sideways, keeping your arms parallel to each other with your right arm beside your ear.

9. Keep your left arm at shoulder height as you transfer your weight onto your right leg and straighten your left leg.

10. Open your right arm in a sweeping motion to the right side as if you are drawing a semi-circle, bending your body forward and bending both knees.

11. Return to the starting position, with both of your legs straight and both of your arms at your sides.

12. It should take you between 20 and 30 seconds to do this sequence.

13. Repeat 4 times before changing sides.

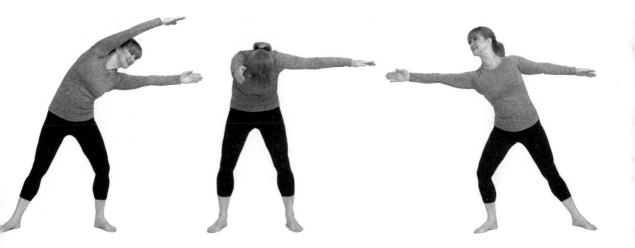

# SINGLE-ARM FIGURE 8

**Use visualization to stimulate your neurons:** Imagine twisting your arm like a corkscrew inside the shoulder joint.

**This sequence will** rebalance muscles around the shoulder joint, through complex rotation within the joint followed by large movement of the full joint. It will release shoulder and neck tension while strengthening the stabilizing muscles around the joint. It is a healing sequence for the upper body and will improve your posture.

**You should be feeling the work** in the shoulder girdle and throughout your back, as your back muscles and sheets of fascia are being stretched.

1. Stand with your legs slightly wider than hip-width distance apart, with your feet comfortably turned out on the floor. The degree of safe turnout varies from person to person. With the correct foot placement, you shouldn't feel any stress in your hips, knees, or feet. Adjust your feet accordingly and choose what degree of turnout works best for you.

2. Bend your knees.

3. Raise your left arm, keeping your right arm at your side.

4. Twist your left arm, like a corkscrew, within the shoulder joint and tuck your tailbone under to create the C-shape of Neutral C. Twisting forces your shoulders to round, and by tucking your tailbone, you will offset the shift of your load path.

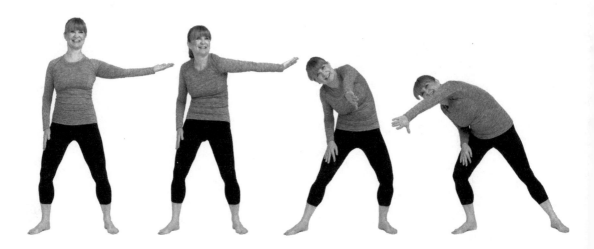

5. Keeping both shoulders facing the front, sweep your left arm directly in front of you, bending your knees and tucking your tailbone under even more.

6. Sweep the arm across the body as far as you can to the right side while bending your body sideways.

7. Shift your weight onto a bent right leg, straightening the left leg.

8. Lift your arm, pulling it as much as possible. Imagine you are trying to touch the ceiling. Drop your right shoulder as you relax your torso, enabling you to lift your arm higher. This will stretch the entire left side of your latissimus dorsi and spine.

9. Straighten your knees.

10. Shift your weight onto a bent left leg, straightening the right and bending your left arm back toward the wall behind you. Try not to turn your torso at first. After 5 seconds, twist your torso and your arm as far as possible.

11. Return to the starting position.

12. This sequence should take 30 to 40 seconds.

13. Repeat 4 times before changing arms.

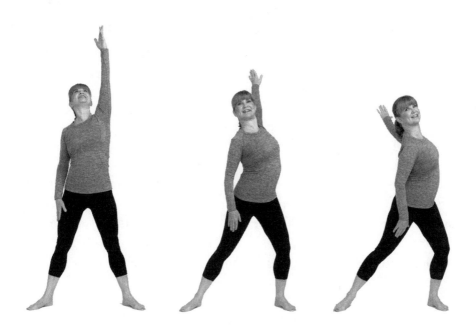

# EMBRACE YOURSELF

**Use visualization to stimulate your neurons:** Imagine comforting yourself as you wrap your arms around your body and rock gently side to side. When you reach upward in a gentle sweep, try to feel a release of negativity from your body and experience the joyful feeling of liberation.

**This sequence will** stretch the fascia of the entire torso, relieving many different pressure points of pain while improving posture.

**You should be feeling the work** in your upper back, hips, and spine.

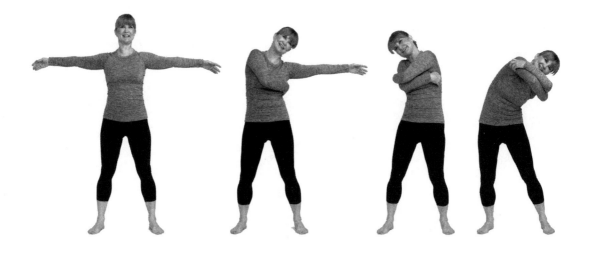

1. Stand with your feet comfortably wider than hip-width distance apart and both arms extended out at your sides.

2. Bend your knees, wrap one arm around yourself, trying to touch the opposite shoulder blade. Repeat with the other arm.

3. Stay in this position and slowly shift your weight from side to side as you embrace yourself.

4. Sway from side to side at least 4 times, taking about 4 seconds per sway.

5. Slowly reach toward the ceiling with one arm, relaxing underneath the armpit and pulling the arm more toward the ceiling. As you do so, round your ribs, allowing them to stretch.

6. Raise the opposite arm above your head and reach toward the sky, relaxing your shoulder blades so that there is no tension preventing you from lifting your arm as high as possible.

7. Return both arms to the beginning position and start all over again.

8. One full sequence should take 30 seconds. Repeat at least 3 or 4 times.

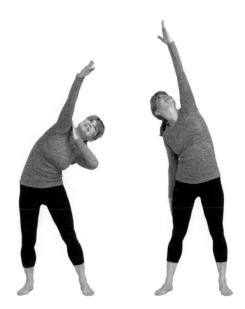

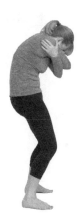

**Side View of Steps 3 and 4**

## HANDS AND ARMS

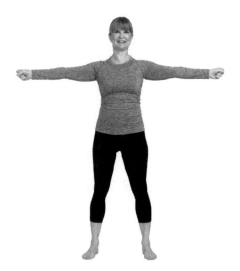

This is the incorrect posture for all of the following arm exercises. Do not shift your hips forward in standing pose. If you lean forward, the spine compensates by shifting the weight backward, resulting in compression of the lumbar region (known as sinking into the spine). This will lead to pain. Other common negative outcomes include arthritis, bulging or slipped discs, and chronic back pain.

# THROWING A BALL

**Use visualization to stimulate your neurons:** Imagine throwing a ball with only the force of your wrists and fingers, not by bending your elbows.

**This sequence will** stretch and strengthen the ligaments and tendons of your wrists and fingers, increasing their mobility. It will also strengthen your forearms.

**You should be feeling the work** in your fingers, forearms, wrists, and shoulders. This is not a pleasant, feel-good exercise. It is tiring, but it is a powerful must-do exercise that will bring you a multitude of anti-aging benefits. Do not skip it unless you feel shooting pain.

1. Start with your legs slightly wider than hip-width distance apart, with your feet comfortably placed on the floor. Some people are more comfortable with their feet slightly turned in and others prefer to have their feet slightly turned out. Choose the position that works best for you. Keep your knees and spine straight.

2. Extend both of your arms to shoulder height with straight elbows.

3. Spread your fingers as wide as you possibly can. Imagine throwing a ball to the floor as you open your hand.

4. Snap the hands into a fist as though you are catching a ball.

5. Repeat 16 times.

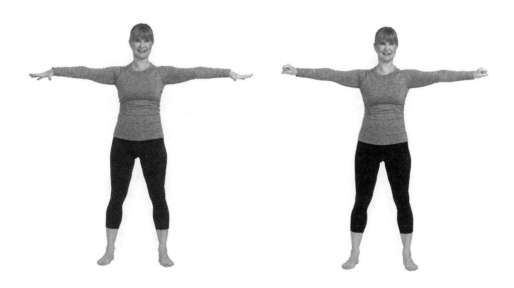

6. Turn your wrists so that your palms are facing the front wall. Imagine throwing a ball to the front wall as you open your hands and snapping them into a fist as you catch it. Repeat 16 times.

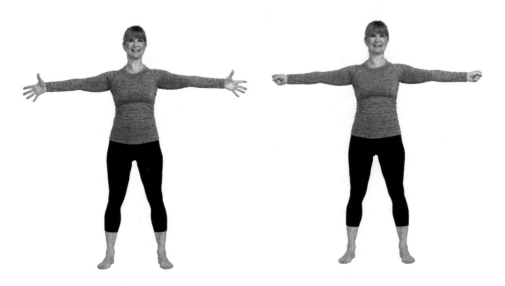

7. Turn your wrists so that your palms are facing the ceiling. Imagine throwing a ball to the ceiling as you open your hands and snapping them into a fist as you catch it. Repeat 16 times.

8. Finish by shaking out your arms.

9. The entire sequence should take you roughly 1 minute.

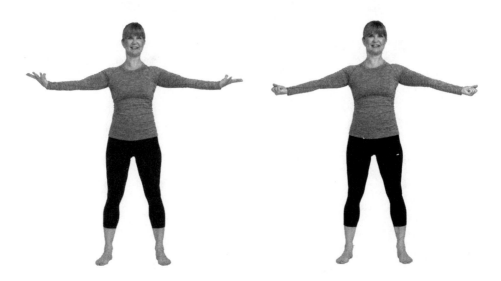

# PUMPING ARMS

**Use visualization to stimulate your neurons:** Imagine pressing your arms down against an invisible force that prevents you from lowering them both rapidly and more than a few inches.

**This sequence will** strengthen and stretch the connective tissue of your underarms, helping to reduce unwanted underarm flab. It helps strengthen the bones of your spine to prevent and reverse osteoporosis and will improve your posture. It lengthens the shoulder girdle muscles, giving you more range of motion in your arms.

**You should be feeling the work** in your shoulders, underarms, and upper back muscles (trapezius).

1. Start with your legs slightly wider than hip-width distance apart, with your feet comfortably placed on the floor. Some people are more comfortable with their feet slightly turned in, and others prefer to have their feet slightly turned out. Choose the position that works best for you. Keep your knees and spine straight.

2. Extend both arms to shoulder height, elbows straight.

3. Slowly pump your arms downward, pushing against an invisible force. Don't let them move more than 3 or 4 inches from their starting position.

4. Repeat 16 times.

5. Slowly pump your arms backward, pushing against an invisible force. This movement will be small. The arms are capable of moving only 2 to 3 inches back from your starting position. Be careful not to let your back move forward into an arched position as you pump the arms back. Hold your core tight to protect your back.

6. Repeat 16 times.

7. Repeat the complete sequence again.

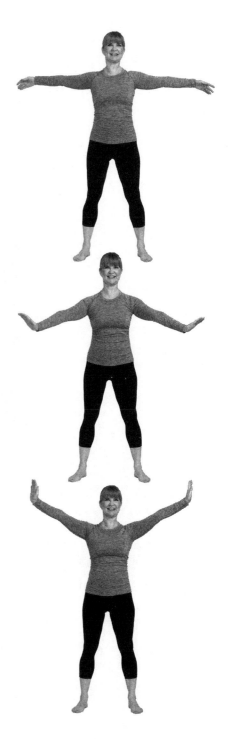

# TRICEPS IN A PRAYER POSITION

**This sequence will** strengthen and stretch the connective tissue around your shoulder girdle and triceps. It is a powerful healing exercise for shoulder and neck pain.

**You should be feeling the work** in your shoulders and triceps and between your shoulder blades.

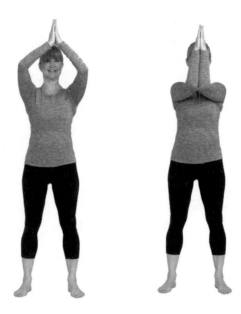

1. Start with your legs slightly wider than hip-width distance apart, with your feet comfortably placed on the floor. Some people are more comfortable with the feet slightly turned in, and others prefer to have their feet slightly turned out. Choose the position that works best for you. Keep your knees and spine straight.

2. Put your palms together in a prayer position above eye level. Do not raise your shoulders.

3. Slowly bring your two elbows together while keeping your arms raised as high as you can.

4. Count 6 seconds as you squeeze the elbows together and then open them to return to the starting position.

5. Repeat 16 times.

# BACKWARD TRICEPS PUMPS

This sequence will tone and strengthen the triceps, which is important for your ability to dress yourself or carry heavy loads such as groceries or suitcases.

You should be feeling the work in your underarms (triceps).

1. Start with your legs slightly wider than hip-width distance apart, with your feet comfortably placed on the floor. Knees are straight.

2. Place your arms at your side with your hands flexed, palms facing the floor and fingers pointing to the front of the room.

3. Imagine that you are slipping your shoulder blades into the back pocket of a pair of pants. Lock the shoulder blades in that position throughout the exercise.

4. Slowly raise your arms backward until you can't lift them higher. From that point, pump them 1 inch up and 1 inch down.

5. Repeat 16 times.

6. Shake out your arms and repeat the full sequence 1 more time.

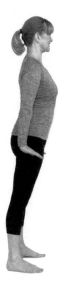
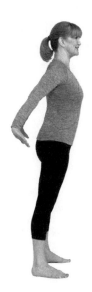
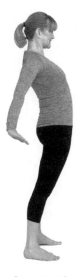

Incorrect

# LARGE ROTATIONS OF THE SHOULDER JOINT

**Use visualization to stimulate your neurons:** Imagine tracing a large circle with the palms of your hands, from the back of the room to the ceiling to the front of the room and back to the floor.

**This sequence will** increase mobility and restore range of motion in your shoulder joint by increasing hydration to the fascia and rebalancing all of the connective tissue. It will reduce various types of pain related to the shoulder joint.

**You should be feeling the work** in your triceps, pectorals, and deltoids.

1. Start with your legs slightly wider than hip-width distance apart, with your feet comfortably placed on the floor. Knees and spine are straight.

2. Extend both of your arms to shoulder height with straight elbows.

3. Flex your wrists, keeping your fingers as straight as you can. Try not to bend your fingers.

4. Trace a large circle with the palms of your hands, from the back of the room to the ceiling to the front of the room and back to the floor. As you draw the circle with your palms, focus on keeping your wrists flexed during the entire sequence.

5. Repeat 4 times in one direction before changing direction, taking 1 minute to draw each set of 4 circles. The complete sequence should take 2 minutes.

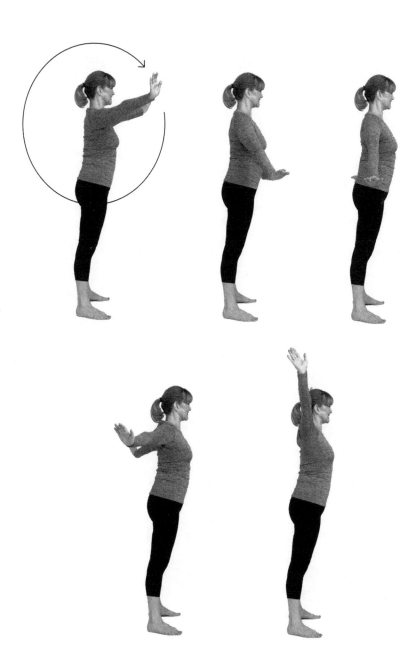

Remember, the chair is meant only to prevent you from losing your balance. Do not grip it tightly, bend forward over it, or hold onto it for dear life.

### FEET AND CALVES

# TOE AND ANKLE ISOLATION WORK

**Use visualization to stimulate your neurons:** Imagine your toes stretching like the wide, webbed foot of a frog.

**This sequence will** increase your energy and relieve pain and injury throughout your body. The ligaments of the toes are connected from the tips of your toes to the top of your skull. When your toes cannot move due to hardened connective tissue, the repercussions of this immobility are felt throughout the body, resulting in stiffness, pain, and potential injuries.

**You should be feeling the work** in your toes, feet, calves, and shins.

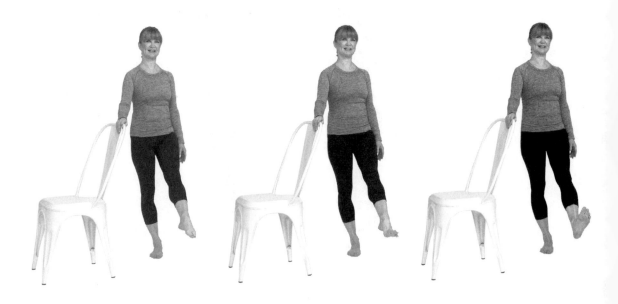

1. Stand next to your chair, placing it slightly in front of your body. Hold the chair with your right hand. Stand close enough to the chair to enable you to keep your arm bent and relaxed. Relax your left arm at your side. Feet are parallel to each other and knees are straight.

2. Maintaining both hips at equal height, extend your left leg in front. Make sure you do not raise the hip of the extended leg. Keep both knees straight.

3. Point your toes as much as you can. Count to 5, continuing to point harder with each count.

4. Slowly flex the toes, stretching them as much as possible. Count to 5, stretching the toes farther with each count. Move only your toes. Do not flex the ankle at all.

5. After you have flexed your toes as much as possible, slowly flex the ankle to its maximum, taking a minimum of 5 seconds.

6. Reverse the exercise by extending the ankles and keeping the toes flexed. Count to 5.

7. Point your toes to their maximum. Count to 5.

8. Repeat the complete sequence 8 times per foot.

# SHIN STRETCH LEVEL 1

**Use visualization to stimulate your neurons:** Imagine you are dropping a carpenter's plumb line from the middle of your kneecap through the center of the arch of your foot. This visualization is designed to help you easily find the perfect skeletal alignment between your ankle and knees.

**This sequence will** stretch the shin and calf muscles, increasing the mobility of the ankle, making walking, running, and climbing stairs easy. Through clean alignment, it will strengthen the ankle ligaments.

**You should be feeling the work** in your ankles, calves, and shins.

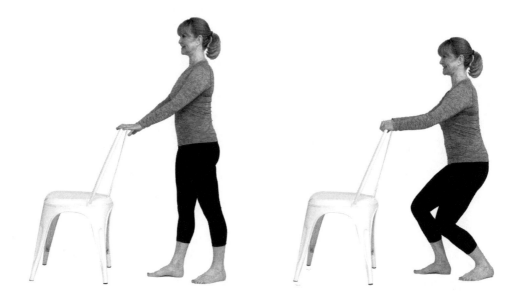

1. Stand facing the back of your chair, holding the chair with both hands.
2. Place one foot in front of the other, with a distance of about 6 to 10 inches between the toes of one foot and the heel of the other. The distance depends on how tall or short you are; taller people need more space, shorter people need less. Adjust according to your own body.
3. Keep your back and legs straight.
4. Bend both knees, making sure your heels are flat on the ground.

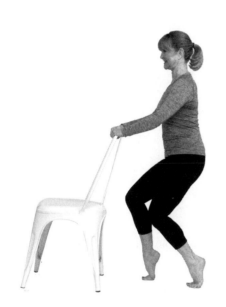 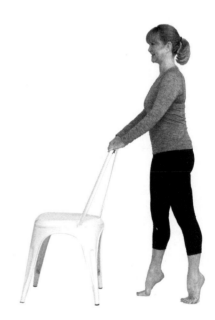

5. Take 5 counts to lift the heels while keeping a clean line (alignment) running from the center of your kneecap, down through your shinbone and the arch of your foot.

6. Take 5 counts to straighten both legs.

7. Take 5 counts to lower your heels.

8. Bend your knees and repeat the sequence 4 times before switching the placement of your feet.

# SHIN, ANKLE, AND QUAD SEQUENCE (SHIN STRETCH LEVEL 2)

**This sequence will** stretch your lower leg muscles, strengthen your ankle ligaments and muscles, and increase the flexibility of your ankles.

**You should be feeling the work** in your shins and arches.

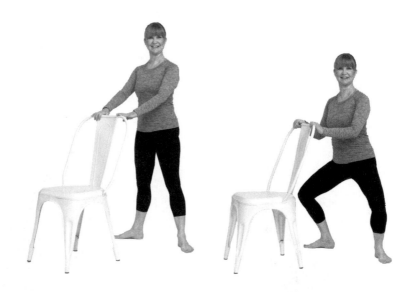

1. Stand facing the back of your chair, holding the chair with both hands. Make sure that the back of the chair is high enough to keep you from having to bend forward.

2. Stand with your feet placed apart at a distance roughly the size of two and half of your own feet.

3. Your feet should be comfortably placed on the floor. Some people are more comfortable with the feet slightly turned in, and others prefer to have their feet slightly turned out. Choose the position that works best for you.

4. Bend your knees as much as you can without triggering any knee pain. Count to 5.

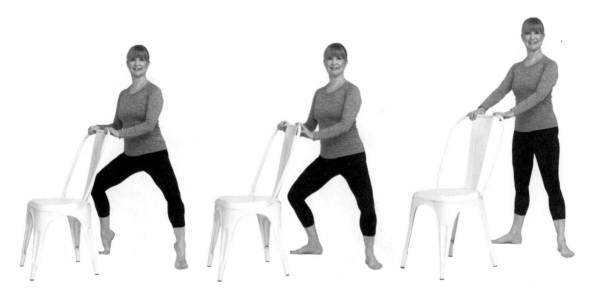

5. Take 5 slow counts to raise your heels while keeping a clean line (alignment) running through the arch of your foot straight up your shinbone.

6. Take 5 slow counts to lower the heels to the ground. As you lower your heels, imagine that you are squeezing an orange under your foot. This will make you work slowly while putting pressure on the muscles, further strengthening your muscles.

7. Return to the starting position with straight legs and repeat 3 times.

# CALF SEQUENCE

**Use visualization to stimulate your neurons:** Imagine giving your calf muscles a deep massage as you move. This will prevent you from employing sharp, jerky motions.

**This sequence will** stretch and strengthen equally the two major muscles of your calf, the soleus and gastrocnemius, and increase your ankle flexibility, putting a bounce in your step and giving you more energy as you walk.

**You should be feeling the work** in your calves and Achilles tendon.

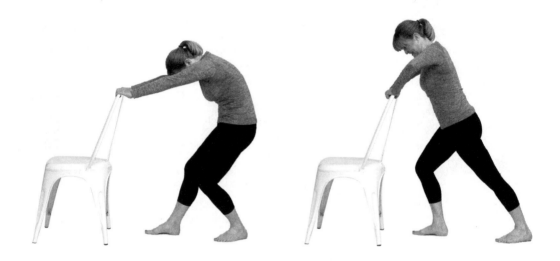

1. Stand facing the back of your chair, holding the chair with both hands.

2. Place one foot in front of the other, with a distance of about 6 to 10 inches between the toes of one foot and the heel of the other. The distance depends on how tall or short you are; taller people need more space, shorter people need less. Adjust according to your own body.

3. Lift your shoulders and round your back. Tuck your tailbone under and lower your head to look at the floor.

4. Shift the weight of your body onto the back leg, with your hips in line with your heel.

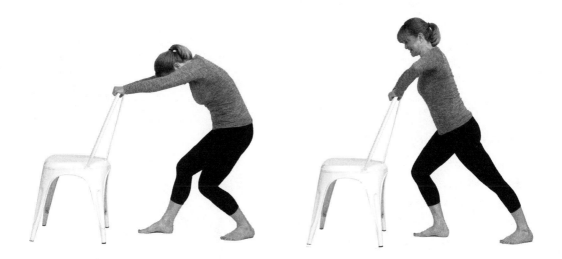

5.  Shift the weight of your body onto the front leg, straightening your spine and lifting your head. Straighten your back leg while digging your heel into the ground. (Do not lift the back heel at all.)

6.  Very, *very* slowly, rock back and forth between the two positions of straight back leg and bent back leg. Your Achilles tendon and soleus muscle are being stretched when the back leg is bent. Your gastrocnemius muscle is being stretched when the back leg is straight.

7.  Repeat 4 times very slowly.

# LIGAMENT PLIABILITY

**Use visualization to stimulate your neurons:** Imagine giving your calf muscles a deep massage as you move. This will prevent you from employing sharp, jerky motions.

**This sequence will** increase the mobility of your ankle joint.

**You should be feeling the work** in your ankles and calves.

1. Stand facing the back of your chair, holding the chair with both hands.
2. Place one foot in front of the other, with a distance of about 6 to 10 inches between the toes of one foot and the heel of the other. The distance depends on how tall or short you are; taller people need more space, shorter people need less. Adjust according to your own body.
3. Counting to 5, slowly raise your back heel, keeping a clean line (alignment) running through the arch of your foot straight up through your shinbone.
4. Round your back and tuck your tailbone under, slightly bending the back knee.
5. Return to the starting position, taking 5 counts as you push the weight of your body through your heel into the floor.
6. Hold the floor with your heel for at least 3 counts before lifting the heel.
7. Raise and lower your heel 4 times before switching legs. It should take between 1 minute and 90 seconds to complete both legs.

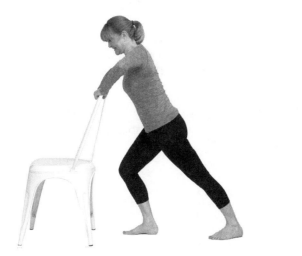
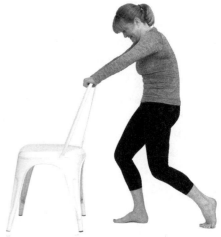

HIPS

# ROTATION WITHIN THE HIP SOCKET

**Use visualization to stimulate your neurons:** Imagine the ball-and-socket joint that connects your thighbone and hipbone. As you rotate your leg, try to feel the rotation *only* within the ball-and-socket joint.

This sequence will be the equivalent to flossing, cleaning out the residue that has accumulated and clogged up your joints.

You should be feeling the work in the hip socket.

1. Stand next to your chair, holding it with your right hand. Extend your right leg in front of you, keeping the knee straight.
2. Flex your right foot, rotating it as far outward as possible.
3. Hold the rotation for 5 seconds, trying to rotate it further.
4. Smoothly rotate the right leg inward.
5. Hold the rotation for 5 seconds, trying to rotate it further.
6. Repeat 8 times before changing legs.

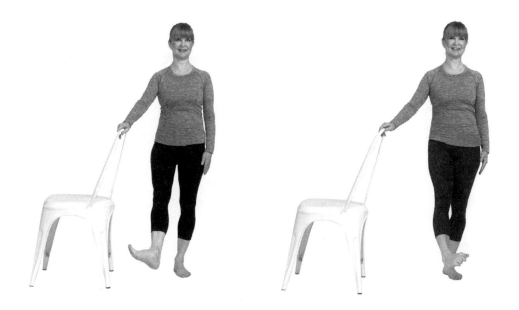

# QUAD STRETCH WITH STRETCH BAND

This sequence will require a stretch band or towel long enough to wrap around your ankle in order to pull your ankle toward your bum without having to bend your back toward your foot.

This sequence will passively stretch your quad muscle, liberating pressure on your knee.

You should be feeling the work in your quadriceps.

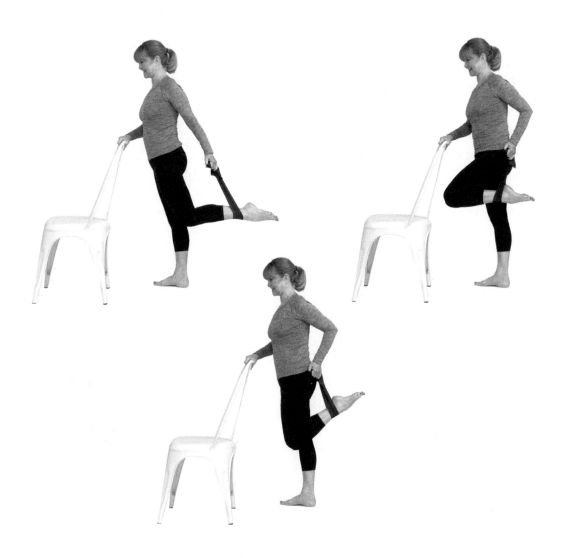

1. Stand facing the back of your chair, holding the chair with your right hand.

2. Stand on your right leg.

3. Using your left hand, wrap your stretch band around the ankle of your left leg, bending your knee and pulling the ankle toward your bum.

4. Without moving your body, swing your bent knee as far forward as possible.

5. Swing your leg back, trying to pull the foot as close to the bum as possible.

6. Swing your leg forward and back 4 times in a slow, relaxed mode.

7. Without moving your back and still holding the stretch band, try to straighten your leg. You should feel tension in your thigh.

8. Relax the effort to straighten your knee and pull the heel as close to your bum as possible, in a very relaxed mode.

9. Repeat this entire sequence 4 times before changing legs.

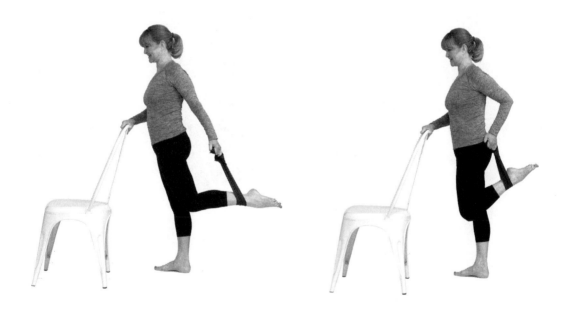

# HIP CLEANER

**Use visualization to stimulate your neurons:** Imagine the ball-and-socket joint that connects your thighbone and hipbone. As you rotate your leg, try to feel the rotation *only* within the ball-and-socket joint.

This sequence will clean out the residue that has accumulated and clogged up your joints and hydrate the fascia in your glutes.

You should be feeling the work in the many muscles of your hip region, including the gluteus group, adductor muscles (inner thigh), IT band, and both hip flexors.

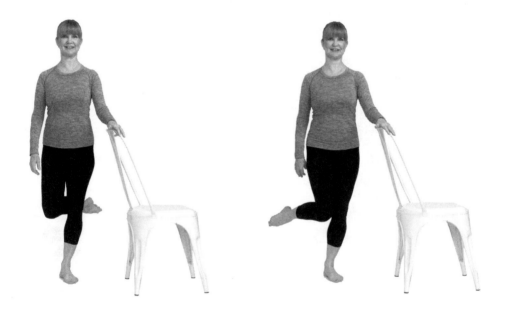

1. Stand next to your chair, holding it with your left hand.

2. Stand on your left leg and raise the right, bending your knee behind you.

3. Keep the bent knee and the standing knee as close to each other as possible.

4. Draw your right heel behind and across your left leg.

5. Keep the two knees together and twist the right leg internally so that your ankle points outward. This will make the thighbone rotate within your hip socket, "cleaning" the hip.

6. Draw the right thigh across the front of your body, lifting it as high as possible.

7. Keeping the right knee bent and the right foot near or touching the left knee, draw the right leg back across the front of your body and open it as wide as possible to the side.

8. Repeat the entire sequence slowly 4 times before changing legs. Each leg should take about 45 seconds.

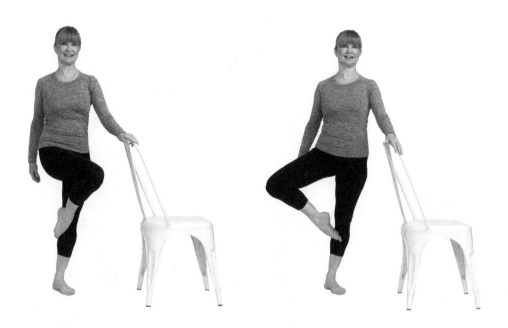

# HIP STRETCHES

**Use visualization to stimulate your neurons:** Imagine your bum swaying side to side and under and back as you move your hips.

**This sequence will** loosen up your lower back and hip muscles, helping to relieve back pain and improve posture.

**You should be feeling the work** in all of your gluteal muscles.

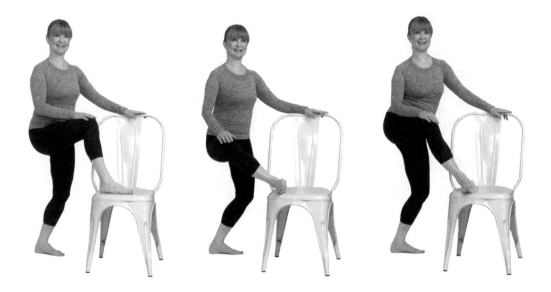

1.  Stand next to your chair, holding it with your left hand.

2.  Place your right foot flat on the seat of the chair, making sure that your whole foot is flat on the seat. You may bend your knee if it hurts to keep it straight. Bend your left leg.

3.  Drop the right knee and the right hip, so that your right hip protrudes outward.

4.  Lift your knee up and rotate it internally toward the seat of the chair and then back down, permitting the bum to sway along with the movement. Repeat slowly 4 times.

5.  End with your right knee open, dropping toward the floor.

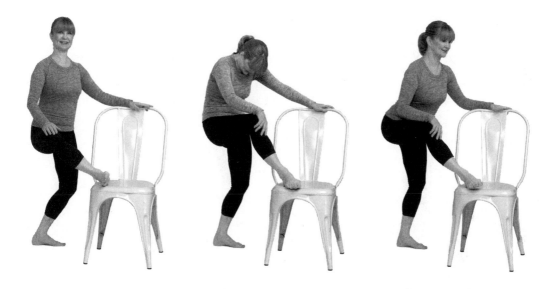

6. Tuck your tailbone under as you round your spine, drop your head, and lift your shoulders.

7. Reverse that spinal position by slowly arching your spine, sticking your bum backward and dropping the shoulders.

8. Repeat the rounding and arching your back motion 4 times before changing legs. Each leg should take about 40 seconds.

# HAMSTRING AND PSOAS STRETCH

This sequence will stretch your hamstrings and your spine.

You should be feeling the work in the front and top of your hip and your hamstrings of the leg on the chair.

1. Stand facing the side of your chair, holding it with your left hand.

2. Place your left foot flat on the seat of the chair, making sure that your whole foot is flat on the seat of the chair.

3. Permit your left leg to bend very slightly as your weight shifts forward, dropping your hip toward the seat of the chair.

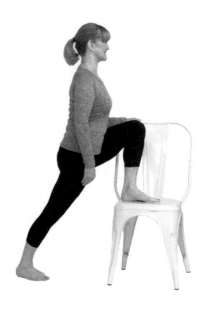

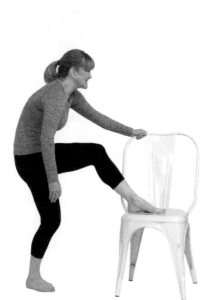

4. Shifting your weight backward onto your right leg, tuck your tailbone under, bend your right leg, and raise your shoulders so that your back is completely rounded.

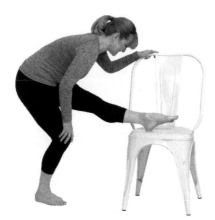

5. Very slowly, try to stick your bum out behind you, as you try to straighten your spine and left leg while pointing the left foot resting on the chair. This movement will pull on your hamstring muscles.

6. Return to the starting position by straightening your right leg and shifting your weight toward the seat of the chair, as you bend the knee. This movement will take the pressure off your hamstring.

7. Repeat 4 times before switching legs. Each sequence should take 30 seconds, for a total of 2 minutes per leg.

# HAMSTRING STRETCH WITH POINTED AND FLEXED FOOT

**Use visualization to stimulate your neurons:** Imagine that you are reaching as far over your leg as possible to touch the opposite wall.

**This sequence will** stretch the hamstrings and the spine.

**You should be feeling the work** in your hamstring muscles.

> This is an extremely deep stretch. Do not force anything. If you cannot do it with a straight leg as shown in the photos, feel free to bend your knee. This will not change the stretching benefits of this exercise; it will just make it safer for you. Never force a stretch or force your body into positions that do not feel comfortable.

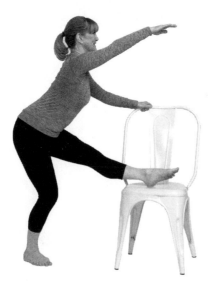 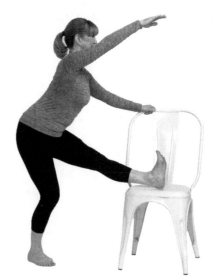

1. Stand facing the side of the chair, holding the back of the chair with your left hand.

2. Place your left foot on the seat of the chair, then point your toe, keeping your knees pointed toward the ceiling. (You may bend your knee if it hurts to keep it straight.)

3. Bend your right leg.

4. Raise your right arm and reach over your left leg, keeping your spine completely straight. Try to keep your spine as straight as possible; this might be challenging if your back is very tight. Never force!

5. *Slowly* flex your left foot. (You will feel a real pull on your hamstrings as you flex your foot, so be sure to flex slowly so as not to overstretch any muscles.)

6. Try not to let your back or bum round during this phase of the stretch; note that many people are incapable of keeping their back straight.

7. Take 5 seconds to point and 5 seconds to flex the foot. Point and flex 8 times before changing legs.

8. Slowly stand up and shake out your body before changing legs.

# HAMSTRING AND SPINE STRETCH WITH ROUNDED TO STRAIGHT BACK

**Use visualization to stimulate your neurons:** Imagine that you are reaching as far over your leg as possible to touch the opposite wall.

**This sequence will** stretch your hamstrings and spine.

**You should be feeling the work** in your hamstrings and spine.

> This is an extremely deep stretch. Do not force anything. If you cannot do it the way I have described it, adjust your body so that it is comfortable. Never force your body in these exercises. Understand that the body will change over time.

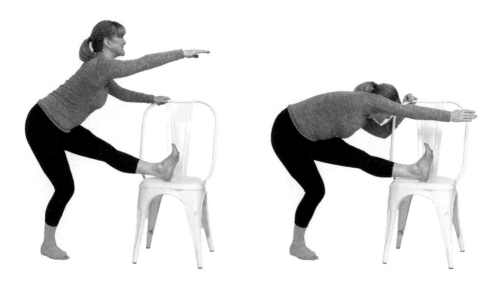

1. Stand facing the side of your chair, holding the back of the chair with your left hand.
2. Place the heel of your left foot on the seat of the chair, flexing your left ankle so that your toes and knee point upward. Keep the left knee as straight as possible.
3. Bend your right leg.

4. Raise your right arm and reach over your left leg, keeping your spine as straight as possible.

5. Draw a semi-circle with your right arm about 2 to 3 inches to the right and to the left. Repeat 4 times.

6. With each small movement of your arm, pull the arm farther toward the opposite wall. As you pull your arm, try to feel it pulling on your spine.

7. Do not let your back or bum round during this phase of the stretch.

8. Round your back and try to lie down on your leg (which you probably won't be able to do). Draw your arm over your leg about 2 to 3 inches to the right and to the left. Repeat 4 times.

9. Slowly stand up, and shake out your body before changing legs.

10. It should take a minimum of 2 minutes for each leg.

# LONG ADDUCTOR AND IT BAND STRETCHES (INNER AND OUTER THIGH)

**Use visualization to stimulate your neurons:** Imagine the ball-and-socket joint that connects your thighbone and hipbone. As you rotate your leg, try to feel the rotation *only* within the ball-and-socket joint.

**This sequence will** rebalance the hip socket by stretching the inner and outer thigh muscles, known as the adductors and abductors. It will also stretch the Tensor Fascia Latae, or IT band, the connective tissue that runs down the length of your outer thigh, in order to liberate the knee and relieve chronic knee pain. A great deal of connective tissue in the hips is loosened and hydrated in these exercises.

**You should be feeling the work** in the inside and outside of your thighs. The IT band stretch is very uncomfortable. As long as you don't force this stretch, do not fear the discomfort.

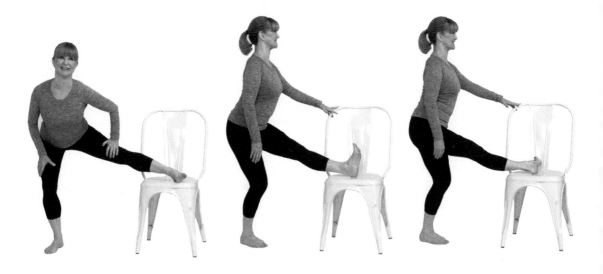

### The Long Adductor (Inner Thigh) Sequence

1. Stand facing the side of your chair.

2. Put your left leg onto the seat of the chair, flexing your ankle so that your toes point toward the ceiling.

3. Bend your right leg.

4. Place your hands on your thighs.

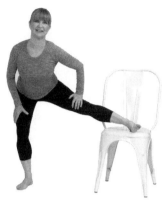

5. Rotate your left leg within the hip socket, letting the foot move like a windshield wiper as the leg rotates. Let the hips lift and lower as much as you want as you are rotating them. Each person feels this stretch at a different point in the rotation of their hip. You will find the place at which your inner leg feels the deepest stretch. When you find that spot, stay there for 5 seconds to deepen the stretch.

6. Repeat the hip rotation 3 times, going from release of the stretch into the deep stretch. This should take 20 seconds per leg.

7. Walk around your chair and repeat this sequence on the other leg.

### The IT Band (Outer Thigh) Sequence

1. Stand facing the side of your chair, holding the back of the chair with your left hand.

2. Place your left leg up on the seat of the chair and bend forward, foot flexed.

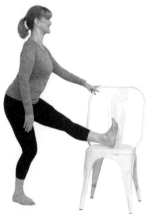

3. Turn the leg outward, rotating within the hip socket, while trying to touch the outer part of your flexed foot to the seat of the chair.

4. Bend slightly sideways toward the left, dropping your left hip. You may find this difficult to do. Do your best and never force.

5. Rotate your left leg within the hip socket, letting the foot move like a windshield wiper going in and out of the deep stretch.

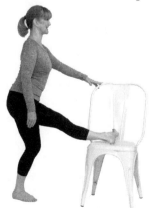

6. Repeat 3 times, taking 10 seconds per repetition, before walking around your chair and repeating this sequence on the other leg.

SPINE

# SPINE STRETCH

**Use visualization to stimulate your neurons:** Imagine that your spine is a stairway and you are going to walk up and down the vertebrae one at a time.

**This sequence will** stretch the spine, relieve back pain, and improve your posture.

**You should be feeling the work** in your hamstrings, spine, and shoulders.

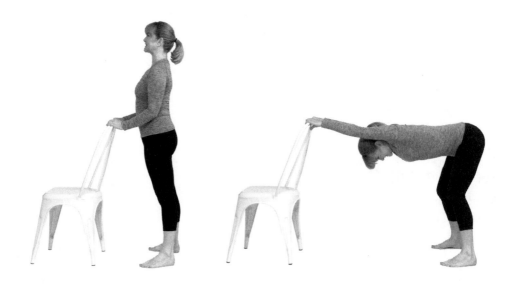

1.  Stand facing the back of your chair, holding the chair with both hands.

2.  Keeping your hands on the back of the chair, walk backward as you bend forward.

3.  Finish with both knees bent, feet wider apart than hip-width distance, arms and spine horizontal with the floor. If you have a very tight spine, you may not be able to straighten your spine to make it horizontal with the floor. Not to worry, do the best you can. In time this exercise will help you straighten your spine.

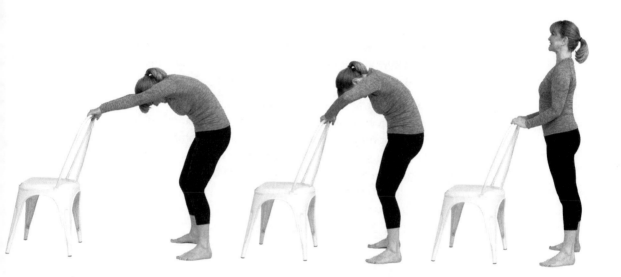

4. Very, *very* slowly, tuck your tailbone under and roll up your spine as you take tiny steps forward.

5. This little walk forward should take about 15 seconds. You want to feel every vertebra as you move toward the chair.

6. This sequence will end in the same position that it began. From start to finish, it should take 30 seconds.

# NECK AND CHEST STRETCH

**Use visualization to stimulate your neurons:** Imagine that you are separating the head from the neck, pulling the vertebrae apart as you stretch the spine upward.

This sequence will liberate tight necks, relieve neck and upper back pain, and reduce headaches.

You should be feeling the work in your neck and shoulder muscles.

- It is extremely important that you do not let your cervical spine (the neck region of the spine) release the upward pull or permit your skull to drop backward. This could compress the vertebra and weaken the neck portion of your spine.

- It will be difficult to tilt your face upward if your neck and shoulder muscles or connective tissue are tight or congealed. Do not try to force higher than you are comfortably capable of. Many people can barely move. That's okay. We are trying to change congealed connective tissue and tight muscles a little bit at a time. The changes may be so minuscule that you won't notice them at first.

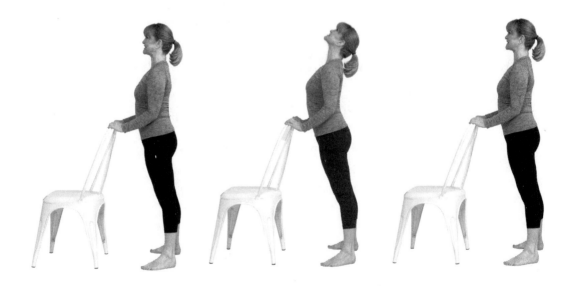

1. Stand facing the back of your chair, holding the chair with both hands. Feet should be hip-width distance apart. Look straight in front of you.

2. Slowly tilt your face toward the ceiling, lifting it upward.

3. As you tilt your head to the ceiling, simultaneously pull your spine upward.

4. Tilt your head back to the starting position, but continue trying to lengthen the spine. Do not release the pull upward on your vertebrae throughout this exercise.

5. Repeat 4 times. Each head tilt should take about 15 seconds from start to finish.

6. Finish by shaking your head and shoulders to relax.

**PART TWO OF WORKOUT 1: Floor Exercises (optional)**

SEATED HIP STRETCHES

# GROIN STRETCH

**Use visualization to stimulate your neurons:** Imagine yourself building up tension in your muscles before deeply releasing and relaxing them, as if they are a rubber ball you can squeeze hard before letting go.

This sequence will release tension in your hips and groin, making all types of movement fluid and easy, such as walking, sitting, dressing yourself, and running.

You should be feeling the work in your hips and groin.

> If you have tight hamstrings or back muscles, sit on a riser.

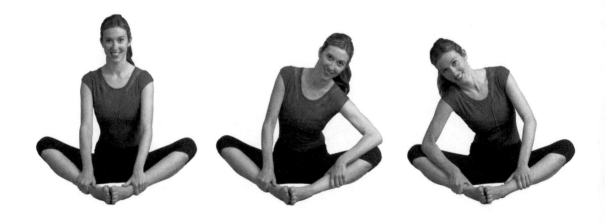

1. Sit with the soles of both feet together, holding your shinbones just above the anklebone. Do not hold your feet. This will result in overstretching and weakening the connective tissue of the ankle joint. Many people mistakenly hold their feet in this position.

2. Bend slightly to the left, placing the left elbow on the left knee. Gently press down on that knee. Hold for 3 seconds.

3. Repeat on the right side.

4. Alternate sides, repeating on each side 4 times.

5. Use all of your leg strength to bring your knees together, while using your arms to prevent you from actually being able to close your legs.

6. Relax the contraction completely, wiggle your hips on the floor, and then relax your bum even more for 6 seconds.

7. Return to the starting position and bend as far forward as you can with your back straight, while your elbows gently push your knees down toward the floor. Let your body relax into this stretch without forcing. Hold for 6 seconds. Some people feel the stretch in their bum and others in their groin. It doesn't matter where you feel it; this depends on which muscle group is the tightest.

8. Repeat the entire sequence 4 times.

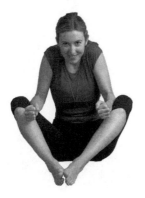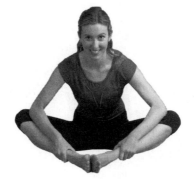

# FIGURE 4 STRETCH

This sequence will release tension in your hips and glutes, relieving back pain and improving posture.

You should be feeling the work in your hips and groin.

> If you have a rounded back that prevents you from maintaining clean alignment when lying on the floor, place a firm cushion under your head. This will straighten the spine and avoid compression in your neck.

1. Lie flat on the ground, knees bent, feet placed flat on the ground hip-width distance apart and arms relaxed at your sides.
2. Breathe deeply 3 times, focusing on relaxing your hips.
3. Bring the right leg up and place the ankle just below the left knee.
4. Wiggle your hips slowly on the floor for 3 seconds.
5. Place the right hand on the right knee and the left hand on the right ankle.

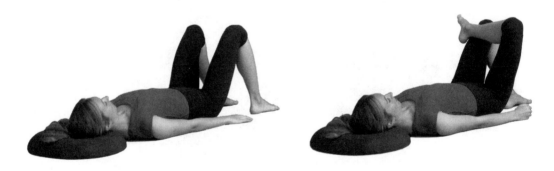

6. Take 4 seconds to lift your left leg off the floor, keeping the knee bent. This will increase the hip stretch on the right side.

7. Shift your hips from side to side, sliding them on the floor, using your hands to help pull the knees in the direction of the shift.

8. Take 3 seconds for each shift of the hips so that you maximize the stretch in that direction.

9. Repeat for 4 shifts before returning to the starting position and changing sides.

10. Repeat the full sequence (both sides) 2 times.

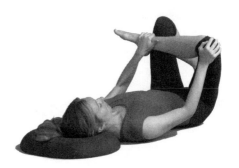

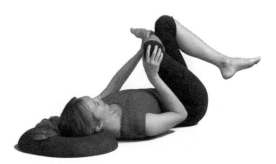

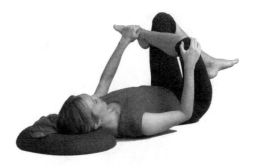

SEATED SPINE STRETCHES

# SEATED SPINAL ROLLS

**This sequence will** release tension in your spine, shoulder blades, and glutes. It will improve your posture and help reduce signs of a dowager's hump. It works deeply through the connective tissue of your entire back, particularly through the shoulders and upper back.

**You should be feeling the work** in your rhomboids, shoulder blades, lower back, hips, and glutes.

> If you have tight hamstrings or back muscles, sit on a riser.

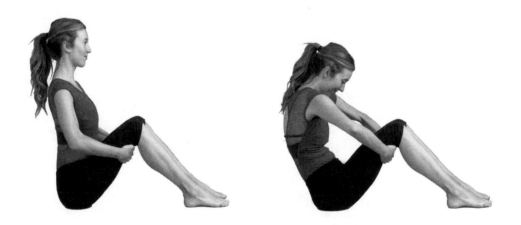

1. Sit on the floor with both of your legs bent, your feet wider than hip-width distance apart and the soles of your feet flat on the floor.

2. Hold your legs behind your knees.

3. Your spine should be straight and pulling upward to the maximum of your ability. Look straight in front of you.

4. Release this position and roll down your spine, one vertebra at a time, rounding your back. This should take 6 seconds.

5. Slowly roll back up one vertebra at a time, maintaining relaxed muscles. This should take 6 seconds.

6. Pull up to your maximum, elongating the spine toward the ceiling. This is the strengthening portion of the exercise and should take 6 seconds.

7. Repeat this sequence 4 times.

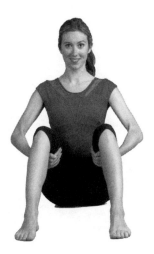

# SEATED SIDE BENDS

**Use visualization to stimulate your neurons:** Imagine that you are following the edge of a large circle on the wall with your fingers.

**This sequence will** release tension in your spine through stretching and strengthening. The combination of this exercise and the previous one will rebalance all of the connective tissue and muscles of your spine, improving your posture and relieving back pain.

**You should be feeling the work** in your ribs, shoulder blades, triceps, lower back, hips, and glutes.

If you have tight hamstrings or back muscles, sit on a riser.

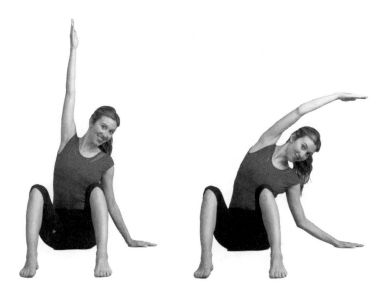

1. Sit on the floor with both of your legs bent, your feet wider than hip-width distance apart, and the soles of your feet flat on the floor.

2. Your spine should be straight and pulling upward to the maximum of your ability. Look straight in front of you.

3. Place your left hand on the floor beside your hip, elbow pointing toward the floor, while stretching your right arm above your head toward the ceiling.

4. Begin to draw a half circle as you bend your torso sideways. Your raised arm should remain close to your ear as you pull it from the ceiling to the wall. This should take 4 seconds.

5. Do not release the tension as you stretch sideways.

6. When you can no longer bend farther sideways, continue the half circle with your torso and arm toward the front of the room. This should take 4 seconds.

7. When you reach the front, with your arm between both legs, stay there and pull farther forward for an additional 4 seconds.

8. Take another 4 seconds to slowly pull your body and arm upright to the starting position.

9. Repeat 2 times before changing sides.

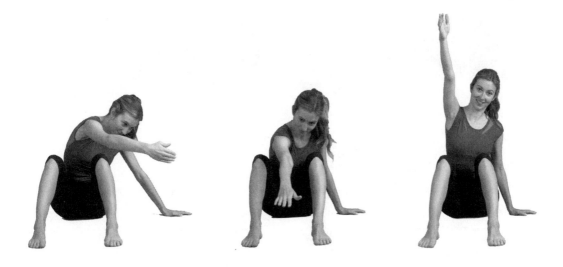

# ROW A BOAT WITH POINTED FEET

**Use visualization to stimulate your neurons:** Imagine that you are rowing a boat with both arms.

**This sequence will** work the large sheets of fascia in your torso, spine, hips, and legs.

**You should be feeling the work** in your back, chest, pectorals, calves, and hamstrings.

> If you have tight hamstrings or back muscles, sit on a riser.

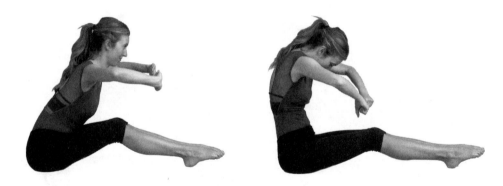

1. Sit on the floor with both legs extended. Slightly bend your knees.

2. Point your feet and pull your spine upward.

3. Raise your arms with bent elbows, lifting upward. The palms of your hands should be facing the front.

4. Imagine you are pushing a weight toward your feet, keeping your back straight as you bend forward. This should take 6 seconds.

5. When you reach your maximum ability to keep your back straight, round your back. Relax with your back rounded and wiggle around for an additional 6 seconds.

6. Round your back and grab the imaginary oars of a rowboat.

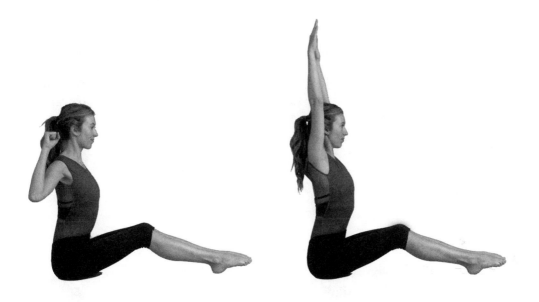

7. Pull the oars back with resistance as though you are really rowing a boat. This should take 6 seconds.

8. When you arrive with your arms close to your ears, do a giant shoulder joint rotation, finishing with your hands beside your shoulders.

9. Extend your arms above your head.

10. Once your elbows have straightened completely, relax your shoulders and pull your arms, spine, and torso, with full strength, toward the ceiling. This should take 6 seconds.

11. Repeat this full sequence 4 times.

DEEP LEG STRETCHES

# HAMSTRING STRETCH

**This sequence will** stretch the connective tissue and muscles of your glutes and hamstrings. It will increase your energy, give you a wider stride as you walk and run, reduce tightness in your back, and improve your posture.

**You should be feeling the work** in your hamstrings and glutes.

- If you have a rounded back that prevents you from maintaining clean alignment in your spine when lying on the floor, use a riser to lift your head up. This will straighten the spine and avoid compression in your neck.

- If you have trouble holding on to your leg without lifting your back off the floor, use a stretch band or a towel to avoid raising your back off the floor and straining your neck. Raising your back also interferes with your ability to release the muscles into a stretch.

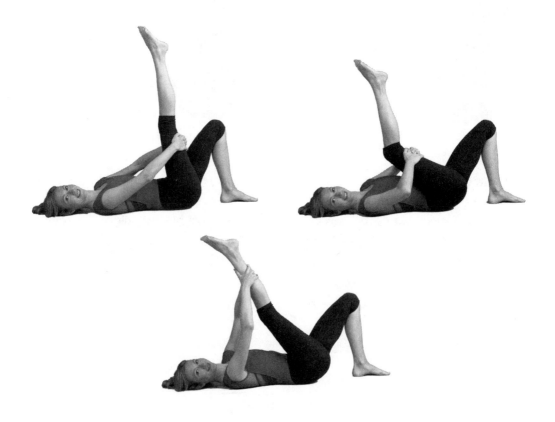

1. Lie flat on the ground, with your left knee bent and the sole of the foot flat on the ground.

2. Raise your right leg with pointed toes.

3. Hold the right leg with both hands beneath the thigh or calf. Use a stretch band or towel if needed.

4. Take 6 seconds to bend the left knee, pulling it toward your chest.

5. Take 6 seconds as you try to straighten the left knee. Most people cannot straighten their knee. You will feel this stretch in your hamstrings.

6. Take 6 seconds to bend the left knee again and pull the left leg toward your chest, while wiggling your bum slowly 4 times.

7. Take 6 seconds as you try again to straighten the left knee.

8. Repeat bending the left knee, wiggling the bum, and straightening the left knee 2 times before changing legs.

9. Repeat the complete sequence on both legs with flexed feet.

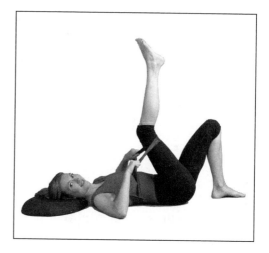

**Optional**

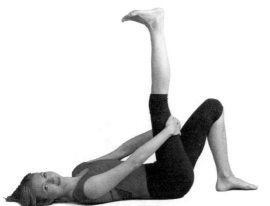

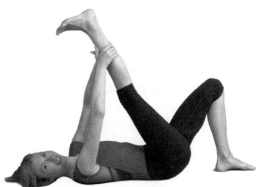

# IT BAND STRETCH

**This sequence will** stretch the IT band, a wide strip of connective tissue that runs down the length of the outer thigh, from the top of the pelvis to the shin. When it becomes tight, it causes arthritis in the knee, chronic knee pain, and possibly the need for knee replacement.

**You should be feeling the work** on the outside of your thigh and hip. You may feel a minor discomfort near your knee. As long as it is not a sharp pain, do not worry.

> If you have tight hamstrings or back muscles, use a stretch band, as seen in the photo on page 233.

1. Lie flat on the ground, with your right knee bent and the sole of the foot flat on the ground.
2. Raise your left leg, foot flexed.
3. Hold the outside of your left leg with your right hand, keeping your left arm flat on the ground.
4. Take 6 seconds to gently pull the left leg across the right side of your body. If you need to use a stretch band or towel, do so.

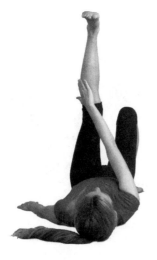

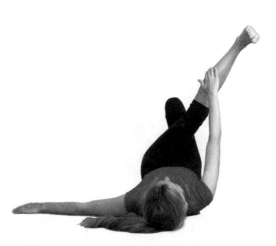

5. Hold this stretch as you inhale for 3 seconds.

6. As you exhale for 3 seconds, try to pull the leg slightly farther down toward the floor.

7. Repeat the breathing sequence 3 times.

8. Return to the starting position and relax your leg muscles by wiggling your leg and your hips.

9. Repeat the complete sequence 3 times before changing legs.

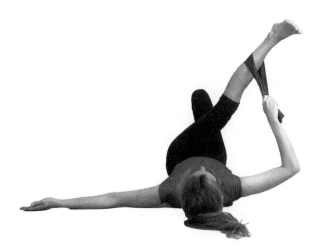

# WORKOUT 2: DAYS 11–20

### PART ONE OF WORKOUT 2: Standing and Chair Exercises

### PART TWO OF WORKOUT 2: Floor Exercises (optional)

**PART ONE OF WORKOUT 2: Standing and Chair Exercises**

## STANDING EXERCISES

**WARM-UP SEQUENCE**

The warm-up involves three different exercises, each of which should be repeated 16 times. When you finish all three, start again from the beginning. Repeat at least twice. Warming up should last a minimum of three minutes. These zero-impact cardiovascular exercises will raise your body temperature by warming up your muscles and releasing tension throughout your full body.

Be sure to maintain a steady deep-breathing pattern throughout your warm-up.

# THROW A FRISBEE

**Use visualization to stimulate your neurons:** Imagine throwing a Frisbee in an extremely relaxed and slow-motion mode.

**This sequence will** increase blood circulation in your full body to warm up the musculature.

**You should be feeling the work** in your thighs, ankles, shoulders, and spine.

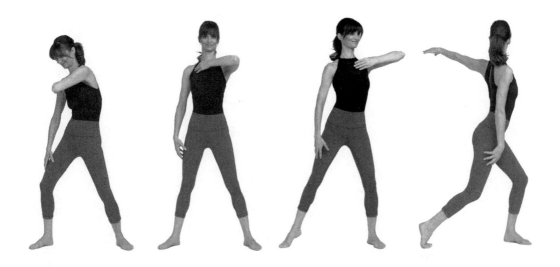

1. Stand with your feet wider than hip-width distance apart. Bend your knees.

2. Relax your right arm at your side, while touching your right shoulder with your left hand.

3. Relax your upper body and twist it slightly to the right.

4. Straighten your back and knees, while coming to the center.

5. Shift your weight onto the left leg, bend both of your knees, and wipe your hand across your collarbone as you draw your arm across your body and twist toward the other side of the room. Imagine throwing a Frisbee. Let the body relax as it twists. Remember, do not use momentum. Proceed in a medium to slow-motion mode.

6. Return to the starting position.

7. Repeat 8 times before switching sides.

# DIAGONAL TWISTS

**Use visualization to stimulate your neurons:** imagine twisting around your spine as though it is a corkscrew.

**This sequence will** warm up all of the muscles of your spine while loosening congealed connective tissue. It will also improve posture and prevent back pain.

**You should be feeling the work** in your spine, shoulders, hips, and knees.

1.  Stand with your feet slightly wider than hip-width distance apart, in a comfortable turn-out that starts at your hips. Your turnout starts with the rotation of the hips, not with the placement of your feet.

2.  Bend your knees and elbows while bringing your hands to touch your collarbones. Your elbows are at shoulder height.

3.  Shift onto your right leg, raise your left arm in front of you diagonally and your right arm diagonally behind as you twist on your spine.

4.  Point your left foot.

5.  Return to the starting position, both knees and elbows bent.

6.  Repeat this identical diagonal twist in the other direction. The shift should be very smooth and fluid.

7.  Alternating sides, repeat each side 8 times.

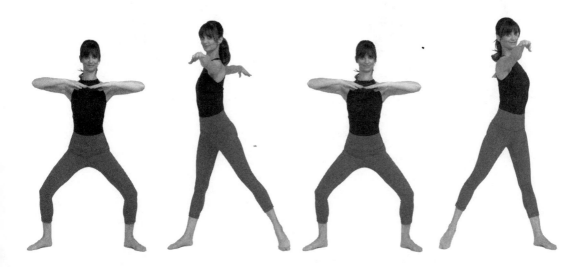

# FULL-BODY ROTATIONS

**Use visualization to stimulate your neurons:** Imagine drawing a full 360-degree circle with both arms starting above your head, moving down toward the floor, and then back up to end above your head. As you bend your spine, imagine the individual 27 vertebrae moving one at a time and not held straight as a rigid rod.

**This sequence will** increase blood circulation in your full body to warm up the musculature. It will lubricate the full connective tissue of your torso, which includes all your joints: shoulders, spine, and hips. It will loosen and unlock tight muscles, which prevent full flexibility of the spine as you move it in every direction it's designed to move in, improving your posture and preventing or reversing spine shrinkage.

**You should be feeling the work** in your shoulders, spine, and ribs.

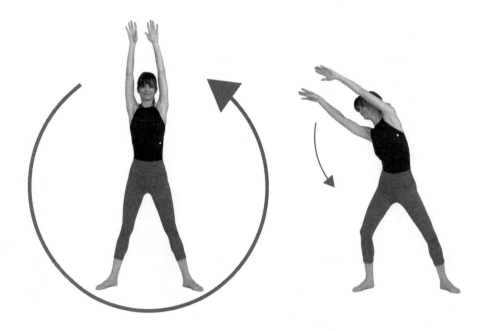

1. Stand with your feet slightly wider than hip-width distance apart and your arms above your head, shoulder-width distance apart. Your spine should be straight. If you can't straighten up, it's okay. Do your best.

2. Keep your hands shoulder-width distance apart throughout the exercise. Don't let your hands move farther apart during the full-body rotation.

3. Slowly bend your entire body sideways, one vertebra at a time. Follow the outline of a 360-degree circle with both arms moving sideways, forward, to the other side, and back up to the starting position.

4. Don't let your arms tighten in the shoulders. Relax the shoulder sockets and pull your arms as far out of the shoulder sockets as possible for the duration of this exercise.

5. One full-body rotation should take 20 seconds. Do not go any faster.

6. Repeat 3 times on each side.

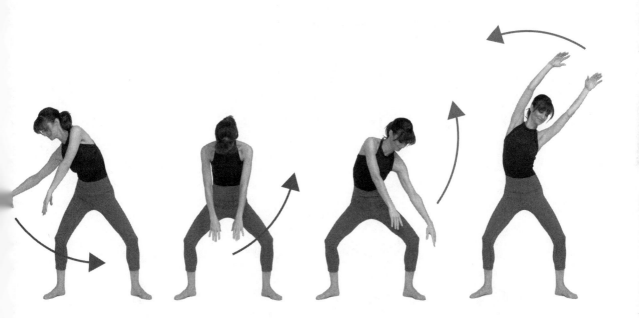

TRADEMARK SEQUENCE

# SPINAL ROLL WITH CEILING REACHES

**Use visualization to stimulate your neurons:** Imagine your spine as a bicycle chain, rolling up one link at a time, starting at the base and finishing at the top.

**This sequence will** prevent and relieve back pain while improving your posture by loosening and hydrating the sheets of connective tissue in your entire back. It will also stretch and strengthen all of the muscles and ligaments that support the spine. In doing so, you will build the fibers of the crimp that are essential to support your spine and maintain good posture.

**You should be feeling the work** in your spine, shoulders, pectorals, ribs, and obliques.

> Move slowly the entire time. Don't stop and start or be jerky. Keep the movements flowing.

1. Stand with your feet parallel and comfortably placed on the floor, slightly wider than hip-width distance apart. Do not force your feet to turn in or turn out.

2. Place your hands on your knees as you bend them.

**Front View**

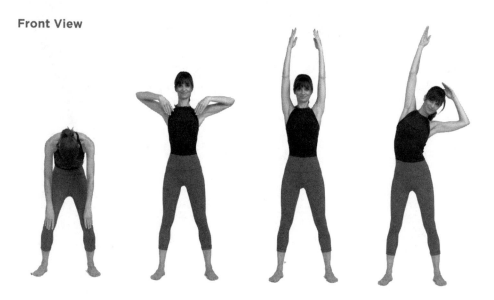

3. Round your spine, making sure that your lower back is as tucked under as possible, and that your shoulders do not drop beyond your knees. Do not stick your bum out or arch your back as this will compress your spine rather than stretch it.

4. Slowly roll up one vertebra at a time, trying to feel each vertebra as it shifts into an elongated spinal position.

5. As you are rolling up, follow your body with your hands.

6. When your hands reach shoulder height, straighten your knees. Extend your arms over your head, pulling them toward the ceiling while relaxing the shoulder sockets. Do not tense your muscles. By relaxing your shoulders, you will be able to raise your arms higher above your head. Count to 6 as you pull your arms above your head.

7. Relax your left arm and lower your left shoulder while pulling your right arm straight up toward the ceiling for a ceiling reach.

8. You will feel the stretch through your ribs and obliques.

9. Keep pulling your right arm toward the ceiling while you gently pull it behind your ear. Do not arch your back or force your arm beyond its comfort zone. You should feel no pain in this stretch.

10. Repeat this sequence with your left arm. It should take 5 seconds per arm.

11. Return both arms to the center, pulling toward the ceiling.

12. Finish by reversing the spinal roll downward.

13. Repeat this entire sequence 4 times. Each sequence should take at least 40 seconds.

**Side View**

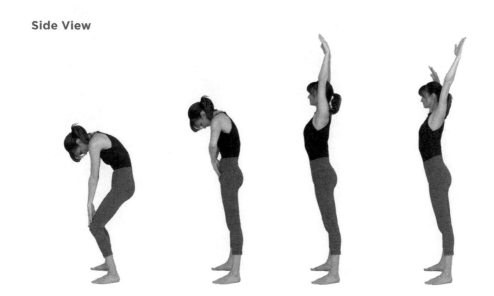

# WAIST ROTATIONS

**Use visualization to stimulate your neurons:** Imagine drawing a circle with your fingertips on the ceiling.

This sequence will lengthen, strengthen, and rebalance your spine in order to relieve or reverse back pain. It will loosen and hydrate the connective tissue throughout your entire back, including fascia, tendons, and ligaments. It will improve your posture and help prevent conditions such as a dowager's hump. It will strengthen the bones of your spine, to relieve symptoms of osteoporosis and reverse shrinkage, helping you regain any height you might have lost.

You should be feeling the work in your spine, rhomboids, shoulders, pectorals, ribs, obliques, and abdominals.

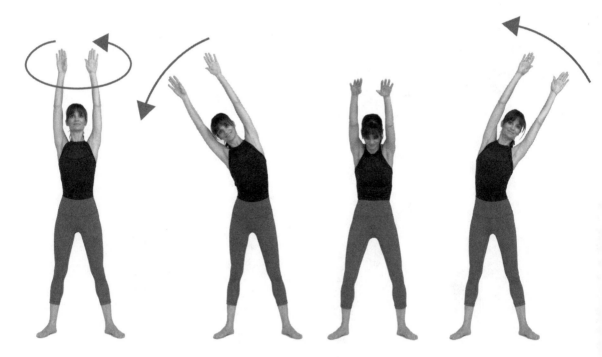

**Front View**

1. Stand with your feet slightly wider than hip-width distance apart, arms pulling upward toward the ceiling.

2. Raise your rib cage so as to slightly arch the upper back. Do not drop your weight, sinking into your lower spine.

3. Bend sideways keeping your spine straight. Imagine that you are beginning to draw a small circle on the ceiling with your fingers.

4. Round your back, bend your knees, and tuck your tailbone under as you draw the circle forward. Straighten your back and knees as you bend to the other side.

5. Slowly finish drawing the circle as you come back to the starting position.

6. One waist rotation should take 20 seconds.

7. Repeat 6 times, alternating directions each time.

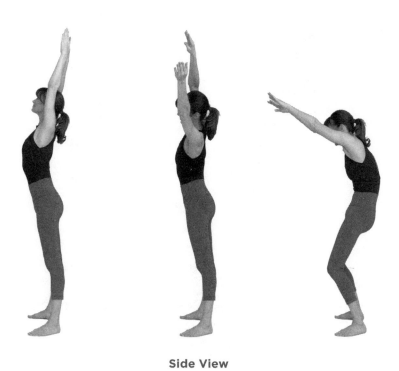

**Side View**

# POLISHING TABLES

**Use visualization to stimulate your neurons:** Imagine polishing a beautiful round antique table using a rag under the palms of your hands to press into the surface. Visualize following the full 360-degree circumference of the table, attempting to reach for the edge.

**This sequence will** increase the flexibility of your spine, helping gain or maintain the full range of motion of all of your individual vertebrae. It will help make everyday movements, such as dressing yourself, effortless. It will stimulate and maintain balance reflexes while strengthening your thighs and hips.

**You should be feeling the work** in your lower spine, hips, quads, and waist.

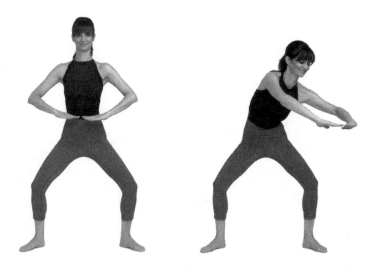

1. Stand with your feet in a wide stance, knees and elbows bent with your palms facing down to the floor at waist height.

2. Keep your knees bent throughout this sequence. Avoid straightening them. If your legs get tired, shake them out and start again.

3. Bend slightly to your left with your palms flat on the imaginary surface of a table.

4. Follow the circumference of the table, from your left side to the front of the table and all the way to the right side, as if you are polishing the top of the table.

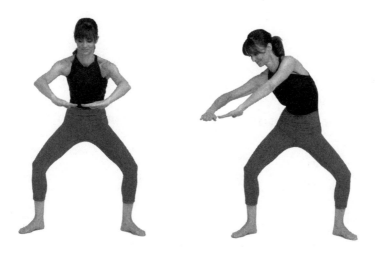

5. Finish in the starting position with a straight back.

6. One table polish should take 15 seconds.

7. Repeat 2 times before changing sides.

8. Repeat this whole sequence a second time, taking a total of 2 minutes.

# WASHING WINDOWS

**Use visualization to stimulate your neurons:** Imagine washing a window at shoulder height, using both arms. Visualize pressing a cleaning cloth against the window with the flat of both hands.

**This sequence will** increase the flexibility of your spine, shoulders, wrists, hips, knees, and ankles. It works through the chains of the body, releasing congealed connective tissue to reverse chronic pain such as as sciatica, back pain, shoulder pain, knee pain, ankle pain, and plantar fasciitis.

**You should be feeling the work** in your shoulders, spine, ribs, hips, and knees.

1. Stand with your legs wide apart.
2. Bend the left leg while keeping the right leg straight. Don't let the bent knee extend over your foot.
3. Lock your hips in place as you bend sideways to the left, raising both of your arms to frame your face.
4. Open your hands, spreading your fingers and imagining that the palms of your hands are lying flat on an imaginary window in front of you.
5. Shift your weight to the right leg as you bend the knee and straighten the left leg.

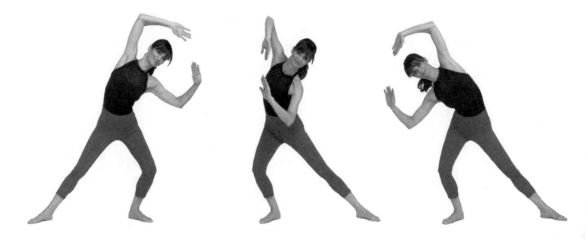

6. As you shift your weight onto the right leg, imagine you are wiping the window in front of you with both hands. Continue wiping the window until you end up in the starting position on the other side.

7. This should take you 15 seconds per side.

8. Alternating sides, repeat 8 times, for a total of 2 minutes.

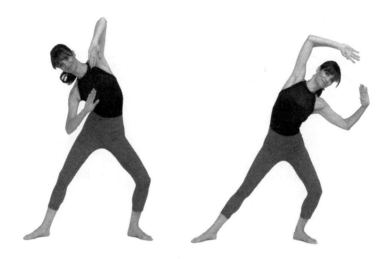

# PUSH THE PIANO AND PULL THE DONKEY

**Use visualization to stimulate your neurons:** Imagine pushing a piano away from your chest and pulling a donkey toward you. When you push the piano or pull the donkey, you can decide how difficult it is to perform these movements. If you work very hard, your muscles will become stronger, whereas if you work in a softer mode, you will increase your flexibility. Either way is good for you.

**This sequence will** strengthen your muscles and increase the flexibility of your spine, shoulders, hips, knees, and ankles. One of the benefits of this large full-body sequence is that it works through the chains of the body, releasing congealed connective tissue to reverse chronic pain.

**You should be feeling the work** in your shoulders, spine, ribs, hips, and knees.

1. Stand in a wide stance with one leg in front of the other and both knees bent, with the weight equally distributed on the front and back leg.

2. Lift your bent elbows upward, in line with your shoulders, the palms of your hands placed flat on an imaginary piano in front of you.

3. Raise your shoulders.

4. Start pushing the imaginary piano, bending the front knee and letting the back leg straighten out.

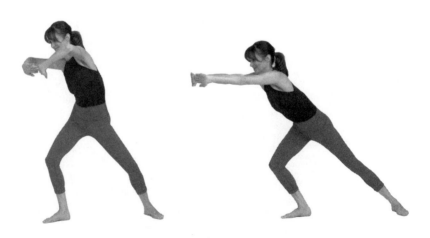

5. Pushing the piano should be slow and take about 10 seconds.

6. Reach a little further to grab an invisible rope attached to the imaginary donkey.

7. Tuck your tailbone under, round your back, and start pulling the donkey toward you as you simultaneously shift your weight onto your back leg, bending the back knee.

8. Pulling the donkey should be slow and take 10 seconds.

9. Repeat 4 times before changing sides.

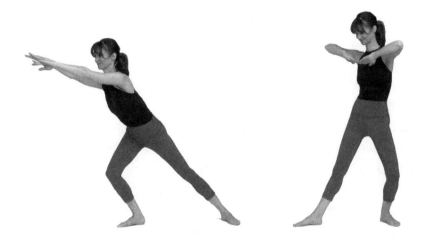

# LULLABY

**Use visualization to stimulate your neurons:** Imagine swaying side to side, as though you are rocking your upper body in a soothing manner to a lullaby.

**This sequence will** increase the flexibility of your shoulders and upper back. It will loosen up congealed connective tissue that often glues the shoulder blades in place, which is a common cause of poor posture, the dowager's hump, and a limited range of motion in the arms.

**You should be feeling the work** in your shoulders, upper back, and shoulder blades.

1. Stand with your feet in a wide stance with bent knees.
2. Keep your knees bent throughout this sequence.
3. Bend your elbows, lifting them to shoulder height. Your palms should be turned away from your face and your elbows should be as close to each other as possible.
4. Bend slightly sideways to your right.
5. Slowly sway your body from side to side, holding your arms in the same position throughout this sequence. Repeat 8 times.
6. Each set of 8 side-to-side sways should take 30 seconds.
7. Shake your arms out and start again.
8. Repeat the full sequence 4 times.

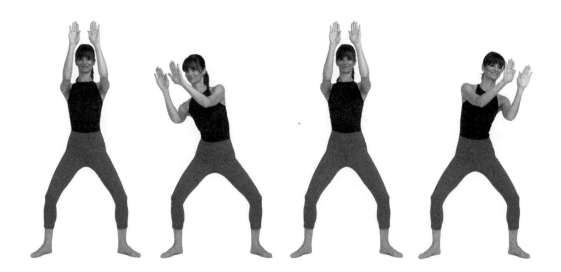

HANDS AND FINGERS

# CATCH A BALL

**Use visualization to stimulate your neurons:** Imagine throwing and catching a tennis ball.

**This sequence will** increase the pliability of your hands and fingers, stretching and strengthening the ligaments of the joints in your hands and fingers. This reverses and prevents arthritis, relieves pain and immobility associated with carpel tunnel syndrome and tennis elbow, and reduces shoulder pain, neck pain, and chronic migraines.

**You should be feeling the work** in your fingers, hands, and forearms.

1. Stand in a wide lunge, with your left leg placed behind and bent and your right leg straight in front.

2. Your back remains straight throughout the exercise while your right arm remains at your side.

3. Raise your left arm so that your elbow is approximately at the same level as your shoulder. Imagine you are holding a tennis ball in your hand, ready to throw it.

4. Throw the ball, keeping your elbow bent, opening your fingers as wide as you can, and shifting your weight forward onto the right leg, bending it.

5. Reverse it by catching the ball, gripping it as tightly as possible.

6. As you throw and catch the ball, shift your weight back and forth accordingly.

7. Repeat throwing and catching 16 times before changing sides.

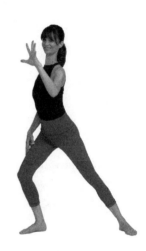

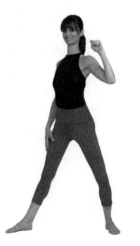

# PLAYING THE PIANO

**Use visualization to stimulate your neurons:** Imagine hitting the keys of a piano with completely straight fingers, one finger at a time including your thumb.

This sequence will increase the pliability of your hands and fingers, stretching and strengthening the ligaments of the joints in your hands and fingers.

**You should be feeling the work** in your fingers, hands, and forearms.

> This exercise feels very uncomfortable in your forearms as the muscles start to contract. Don't worry, the discomfort will disappear the moment you stop.

1. Stand in a wide stance with straight legs and spine.
2. Bend your elbows, keeping your elbows at waist height. Palms face the floor. Stretch your fingers to their maximum.
3. With your thumb held straight, hit an imaginary key of a piano as hard as you can.
4. Repeat with each finger, going from thumb to pinkie, 16 times. Shake out your hands if they get tired.
5. Repeat the entire sequence with bent fingers 16 times.

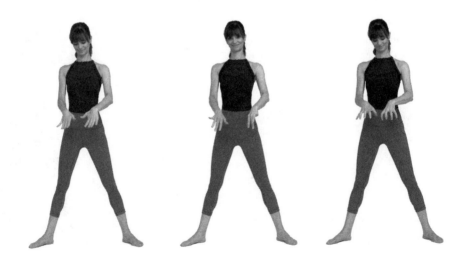

HIPS AND LEGS

# CALF SEQUENCE

**Use visualization to stimulate your neurons:** Imagine gripping the muscles of your calf so tightly that you can stop the circulation. Releasing the grip rapidly will force the blood to rush into your relaxed calves.

**This sequence will** increase the mobility of your ankles and knees by stretching the two main muscle groups of your calves, your soleus and gastrocnemius. The soleus is a muscle that attaches your foot to your lower leg, while your gastrocnemius attaches your foot to your thighbone. These two muscles must be equally and simultaneously stretched and strengthened in order to have any pain-relief or mobility benefits. A lack of mobility in these muscles may result in the need for knee and hip replacements, plantar fasciitis, and arthritis.

**You should be feeling the work** in your calves and Achilles tendon.

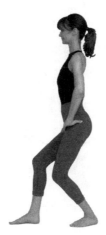

1. Stand with your right foot in front of your left foot with a distance of about 6 inches separating the two feet.
2. Your feet should be hip-width distance apart.
3. Bend both knees. Imagine you are sitting on your left heel when you bend your knees.
4. Hold your hips with your hands.
5. Keep your back pulled-up and straight.

6. Grip your left calf muscle, keeping the knee bent, for 6 seconds. You will be working your soleus muscle.

7. Release the tension and bend your left knee further (you will be capable of bending further).

8. Repeat 3 times.

9. Straighten the left leg, digging the heel into the floor. Don't release the heel from the floor, even the tiniest bit.

10. Grip your left calf muscle, keeping the knee straight, for 6 seconds. You will be working your gastrocnemius muscle.

11. Release the tension as you stretch your left leg further.

12. Repeat 3 times.

13. Change sides and complete the entire sequence again.

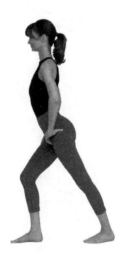

# ANKLE LIGAMENT AND TENDON ALIGNMENT

Use visualization to stimulate your neurons: Imagine that your back heel raises and lowers in perfect alignment with your shinbone. Be very aware not to let the ankle roll either internally or externally. Picture your shin and foot pinned between two panes of glass in order to maintain perfect alignment as your heel moves up and down.

This sequence will retrain and realign the fibers of your connective tissue to restore lost mobility of your ankle joint. This is a pliability exercise, not a flexibility exercise: think only about mobility, not about flexibility.

You should be feeling the work in your calves and Achilles tendon.

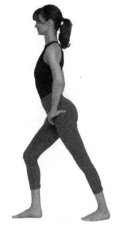

1. Stand with your right foot in front of your left foot with a distance of about 12 inches separating the two feet.
2. Your feet should be hip-width distance apart.
3. Bend your right knee and straighten your left leg.
4. Hold your hips with your hands.
5. Keep your back pulled up and straight.
6. Raise your left heel, keeping it completely aligned with your shin. Make sure that your big toe and second toe remain flat on the floor.
7. Very slowly, take 6 seconds to force the left heel into the ground.
8. Lift and lower the left heel 6 times before changing feet.

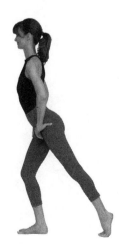

# PSOAS AND QUAD STRETCHES

**Use visualization to stimulate your neurons:** Imagine your hips as a wheel that you are continuously turning in order to round the lower spine.

**This sequence will** relieve back pain by rebalancing the muscles and connective tissue of the hip flexor group composed of your psoas and quadriceps. This muscle group is known for causing back pain and stiffness when imbalanced. Stretching the psoas muscle will improve posture.

**You should be feeling the work** in the front of your hip and in your quads.

1. Stand with your right foot in front of your left foot with a distance of about 12 inches separating the two feet.

2. Your feet should be hip-width distance apart.

3. Bend your right knee and straighten your left leg.

4. Hold your hips with your hands.

5. Keep your back pulled up and straight.

6. Think of your hips as a wheel that you are rotating until you can't tuck your tailbone any further.

7. Lock the tailbone in place and try to straighten your left leg, counting to 4. If you lock your tailbone tight enough in its tucked-under position, it should be impossible to put your heel flat on the floor. You should feel a stretch in the front of your right hip. This stretches the psoas muscle group.

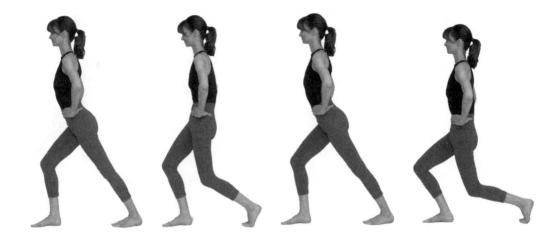

8.  Lift your left heel, bend your knee as much as possible, and tuck your tailbone under, thinking of the hip rotating as a wheel.

9.  Slowly lower your left knee toward the floor. Your thigh should be at a right angle to the floor, with your knee pointed directly at the floor. You should feel a stretch in your quads.

10. Lower the left knee toward the floor as much as you can before feeling pain. The moment you reach your maximum quad stretch, return immediately to the starting position. Do not hold or remain in the stretch; holding the stretch will have the opposite effect by tightening your muscles.

11. Repeat 3 times on each leg. This should take you 1 minute per side.

Remember, the chair is meant to prevent you from losing your balance. Do not grip it tightly or bend forward over it.

FEET

# FOOT PLIABILITY AND ALIGNMENT

**Use visualization to stimulate your neurons:** Imagine the skeleton of your foot. You have 28 bones in your foot, all attached at joints. Each has to move separately in order to maintain healthy foot and full-body alignment. As you do these exercises, picture your joints moving individually and not as an immobile block.

This exercise will increase the health and mobility of the ligaments, tendons, and muscles of your feet. In doing so, it will improve the alignment of your skeleton, starting from your feet and right up into your spine. By liberating your feet and improving mobility, you are starting the process of improving your posture and relieving conditions of arthritis in your feet, knees, and hips. These are massively important exercises as the feet are the foundation of your entire body and they govern your balance. Do not underestimate the value of these simple feet exercises. When your feet are poorly aligned or weak, your body is prone to suffer from joint pain, arthritis, the need for joint replacements, and poor posture.

**You should be feeling the work** in your toes, ankles, shins, and calves.

1. Stand diagonally behind your chair, holding it with your right hand. Your left hand is on your hip.
2. Place your right foot in front of your left foot with a distance of about 6 inches separating the two feet.
3. Your feet should be hip-width distance apart.
4. Bend both of your knees equally with the weight of your body on the back left leg.
5. Keep your back pulled up and straight.
6. Lift your right heel as high as you can, leaving the ball of your foot and the first 3 toes flat on the floor, trying to feel a stretch in the arch of your foot.
7. Point your toes, trying to increase the point for a total of 4 seconds.

8. Flex your foot, trying to increase the flex for a total of 4 seconds.

9. Reverse the exercise: point the foot, return the toes to the floor with the heel raised, and press the heel flat into the floor.

10. Repeat 4 times.

11. Walk to the other side of the chair and do the other foot.

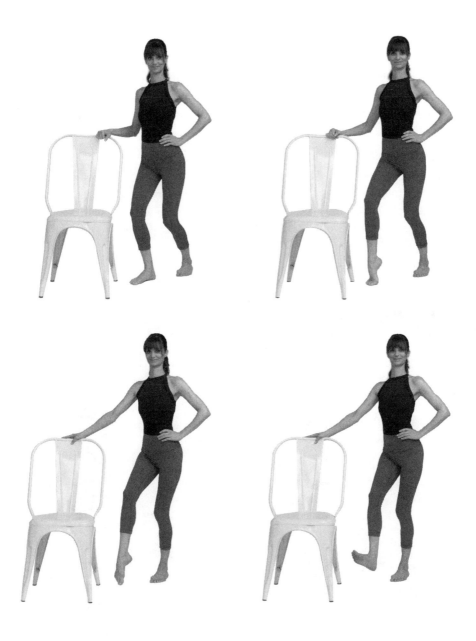

# TOE AND HEEL TAPS

**Use visualization to stimulate your neurons:** Imagine that you are tapping a drum with your toes and then with your heels. The movement should have a light rebound action with each tap.

**This exercise will** stretch and strengthen the hips, increasing the mobility of the hip socket. It will improve your posture.

**You should be feeling the work** in your hips, hamstrings, and psoas.

1. Stand diagonally behind your chair, holding it with your right hand. Your left hand is on your hip.

2. Extend your right leg in front, toes pointed. Both legs should be straight.

3. Your back should be erect with perfect posture. Make sure you do not round your back or tuck your tailbone under. Throughout this exercise, make sure you do not engage your back. It is essential that you isolate the movement of your leg within the hip socket, keeping the rest of the body still. This requires a lot of strength and flexibility of the glutes.

4. Tap the floor 8 times with the toes of your pointed foot.

5. Flex your foot and repeat 8 times, tapping with the heel.

6. Repeat this sequence 4 times (32 taps) before changing legs.

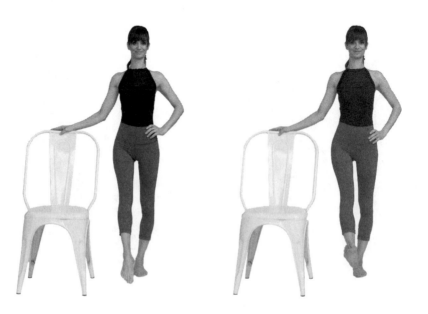

HIPS AND LEGS

# ROTATION WITHIN THE HIP SOCKET

This exercise appears in Workout 1. It is repeated in Workout 2 because it is so effective at releasing connective tissue.

**Use visualization to stimulate your neurons:** Imagine the ball joint of your thighbone moving in the socket joint of your hipbone. This joint is called a ball-and-socket joint because it gives a rotational movement to the leg within the hip. When you rotate the leg internally and externally, imagine your foot as a windshield wiper wiping a window back and forth.

**This exercise will** loosen any debris caused from hardened mineral or connective tissue deposits that make us stiff and limit movement.

**You should be feeling the work** in your hips.

1. Stand next to your chair, holding it with your right hand. Extend your right leg in front of you, keeping the knee straight.

2. Flex your right foot, rotating it as far outward as possible.

3. Hold the rotation for 5 seconds, trying to rotate it farther.

4. Smoothly rotate the right leg inward.

5. Hold the rotation for 5 seconds, trying to rotate it farther.

6. Repeat 8 times before changing legs.

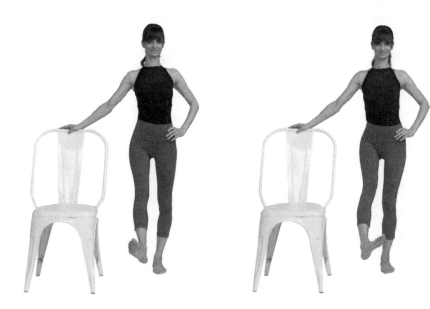

# SPRING KICKS

**Use visualization to stimulate your neurons:** Imagine pushing down on a spring with your foot; when you release the pressure, the spring rebounds, helping you kick your leg upward and shift your weight back.

**This exercise will** strengthen your feet, increase mobility in your ankles, stimulate your balance reflexes, and improve alignment in your feet, knees, and spine.

**You should be feeling the work** in your feet, ankles, knees, and hips.

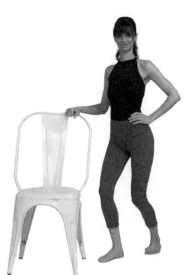

1. Stand diagonally behind your chair, holding it with your right hand. Your left hand is on your hip.

2. Place your right foot in front of your left foot with a distance of about 12 inches separating the two feet.

3. Your feet should be hip-width distance apart.

4. Bend both knees.

5. Keep your back pulled up and straight.

6. Press the full weight of your body onto your right foot, using the knees and thighs, in order to build up pressure under the sole of your foot.

7. Spring your weight back onto the left leg, as you kick the right leg to knee height.

8. Make sure that the entire weight of your body shifts backward so that you are standing completely straight on the back leg, with perfect posture.

9. Do not tuck the tailbone under or raise your hips as you lift the leg in order to isolate the leg within the hip socket.

10. Hold the leg at knee height for 3 seconds, keeping your hips down.

11. With control, return to your starting position.

12. Repeat 16 times per leg.

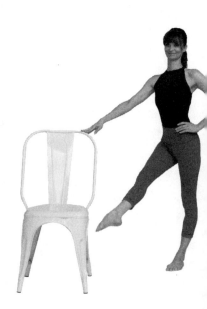

# HIP STRETCHES

**Use visualization to stimulate your neurons:** Imagine rocking your hips in a hammock.

**This sequence will** relieve back pain, increase mobility in the connective tissue of your lower back and hips, and remove any connective tissue debris from the hip socket.

**You should be feeling the work** in your hips.

1. Stand next to your chair, holding it with your right hand.
2. Place your left foot flat on the seat of the chair, making sure that your full foot is flat on the seat. Bend your right leg.
3. Rest your left hand comfortably on your left knee, but don't force your knee to open with your hand.
4. Start rocking your hips from side to side by lifting them up to the left and lowering them down to the floor. Move slowly so that you can go as far as possible in both directions.
5. Repeat the rocking motion 6 times, each time trying to swing your hips a little further.
6. Walk around the chair to the other side and repeat on the other leg.

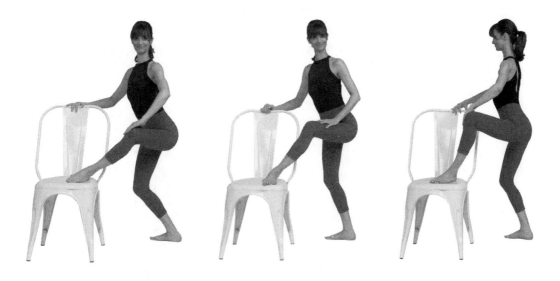

# QUAD STRETCH

**Use visualization to stimulate your neurons:** Think of your hips as a wheel that you are continuously turning in order to round the lower spine.

**This sequence will** relieve knee pain by rebalancing the muscles and connective tissue of the quads.

**You should be feeling the work** in your quads.

1. Stand facing the side of your chair, holding it with your right hand.

2. Place your right foot flat on the seat of the chair, making sure that your full foot is flat on the seat of the chair.

3. Your left leg should be slightly behind you with the heel flat on the ground.

4. Lift the heel of your left leg, bend the knee and slowly lower it toward the floor. You will feel the quad being stretched.

5. Tuck your tailbone under until you can't go any further, thinking of your hips as a wheel you are rotating.

6. Go as far toward the floor as you can with no pain. The moment you reach your maximum, return immediately to the starting position. Do not hold the stretch; holding the stretch will have the effect of tightening your muscles.

7. Repeat 3 times on each leg. This should take you 30 seconds per side.

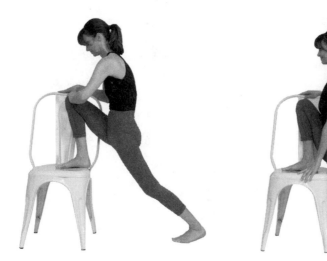

# HIP CLEANER

This exercise appears in Workout 1. It is repeated in Workout 2 because it is so effective at releasing connective tissue.

**Use visualization to stimulate your neurons:** Imagine the ball-and-socket joint that connects your thighbone and hipbone. Rotate your leg and try to feel the rotation taking place within the ball-and-socket joint, and only that.

**This sequence will** be the equivalent of flossing between the teeth by cleaning out deposited minerals that have accumulated and clogged up your joints. As the dentist scrapes away the plaque between our teeth and gums, we are removing the residue between our joints through movement. It will also hydrate the fascia in your glutes, improving its ability to slip and slide.

**You should be feeling the work** in the many muscles of your hip region, including the gluteus group, adductor muscles (inner thigh), IT band, and both hip flexors. ·

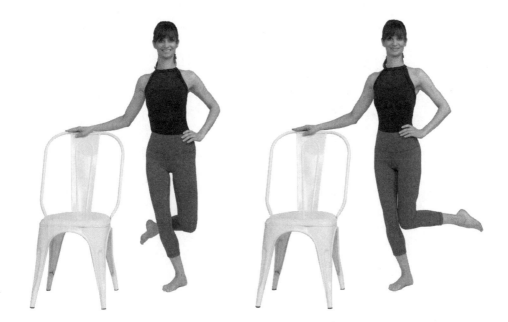

1.  Stand next to your chair, holding it with your right hand.

2.  Stand on your right leg and raise the left, bending your knee behind you.

3.  Keep the bent knee and the standing knee as close to each other as possible.

4. Draw your left heel behind and across your standing leg.

5. Keep the two knees together and twist the left leg internally so that your ankle points outward. This will make the thighbone rotate within your hip socket, "cleaning" the hip.

6. Draw the left thigh across the front of your body, lifting it as high as possible.

7. Keeping the left knee bent and the left foot near or touching the right knee, draw the left leg back across the front of your body and open it as wide as possible to the side.

8. Repeat the entire sequence slowly 4 times before changing legs. Each leg should take about 45 seconds.

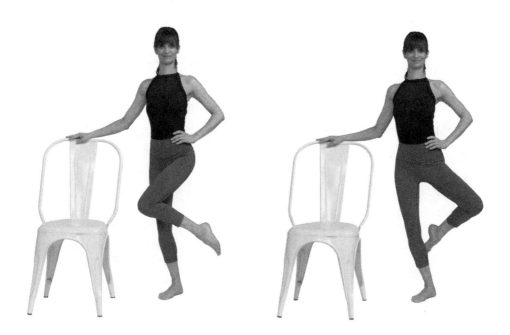

# HAMSTRING STRETCH WITH ARM SWEEPS

**Use visualization to stimulate your neurons:** Imagine your arm sweeping through water in a calm sea.

**This sequence will** relieve back pain and improve posture by rebalancing the muscles and connective tissue of your spine, glutes, and hamstrings. It will also increase the range of motion of your hips, bringing energy and a feeling of effortlessness to movements like walking and running.

**You should be feeling the work** in your back, shoulder blades, glutes, and hamstrings.

1.  Stand on your left leg, comfortably holding the back of the chair with your right arm.
2.  Place your right heel on the seat of the chair with a pointed foot. Make sure you don't lift your right hip while you do this.
3.  Start sweeping your arm from left to right over the leg on the chair. This should be done very slowly so that you can feel individual muscles of your back as they are being stretched. If it is too difficult to keep the knee straight while on the chair, feel free to bend it.
4.  Continue the sweeping motion 4 times before walking to the other side of the chair and changing legs. This is an extremely deep stretch, so shake out your legs before changing legs.
5.  Repeat the entire sequence on both sides with a flexed foot on the chair.

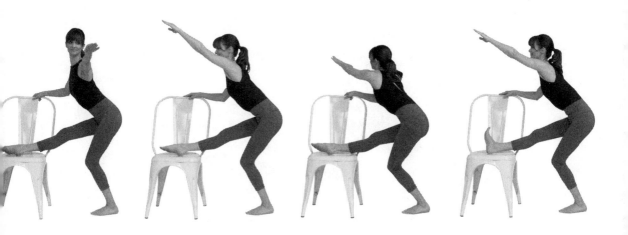

# LONG ADDUCTOR AND IT BAND STRETCHES (INNER AND OUTER THIGH)

Please note that this stretch is similar to the one you did in Workout 1, with subtle but important variations.

**Use visualization to stimulate your neurons:** Imagine the ball-joint of your thighbone moving in the socket joint of your hipbone. This joint is called a ball-and-socket joint because it gives a rotational movement to the leg within the hip. When you rotate the leg internally and externally, imagine your foot as a windshield wiper wiping a window from left to right.

**This sequence will** rebalance the hip socket by stretching the inner and outer thigh muscles known as the adductors and abductors. It will also stretch the Tensor Fascia Latae, also known as the IT band (iliotibial band) in order to liberate the knee, relieving chronic knee pain. A great deal of connective tissue in the hips is loosened and hydrated in these exercises.

**You should be feeling the work** in the inside and outside of your thighs. The IT band stretch is very uncomfortable. As long as you don't force this stretch, do not fear the discomfort.

### The Long Adductor (Inner Thigh) Sequence

1. Stand facing the side of the chair.
2. Put your right leg onto the seat of the chair, flexing your ankle so that your toes point toward the ceiling.

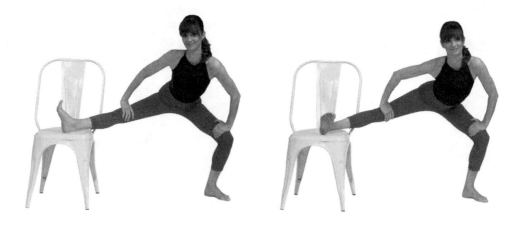

3. Bend your left leg.

4. Place your hands on your thighs.

5. Rotate your right leg within the hip socket, letting the foot move like a windshield wiper as the leg rotates. Let the hips lift and lower as much as you want as you are rotating them. Each person feels this stretch at a different point in the rotation of their hip. You will find the place at which your inner leg feels the deepest stretch. When you find that spot, stay there for 5 seconds to deepen the stretch.

6. Repeat the hip rotation 3 times, going from release of the stretch into the deep stretch. This should take 20 seconds per leg.

7. Walk around your chair and repeat this sequence on the other leg.

### The IT Band (Outer Thigh) Sequence

1. Stand facing the side of your chair, holding the back of the chair with your right hand.

2. Place your left leg up on the seat of the chair and bend forward, foot flexed.

3. Turn the left leg outward, rotating within the hip socket, while trying to touch the outer part of your flexed foot on the seat of the chair.

4. Bend slightly sideways toward the left, dropping your left hip. You may find this difficult to do. Do your best and never force.

5. Rotate your left leg within the hip socket, letting the foot move like a windshield wiper going in and out of the deep stretch.

6. Repeat for a total of 3 times, taking 10 seconds per repetition.

7. Walk around your chair and repeat this sequence on the other leg.

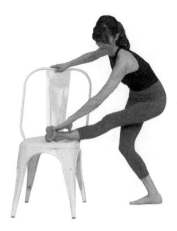

SPINE

# SPINE ROTATION AND SIDE BEND

**Use visualization to stimulate your neurons:** Imagine your spine is a corkscrew in a bottle of wine.

**This sequence will** relieve back pain and improve posture by rebalancing the muscles and connective tissue of your spine. It will also increase the range of motion of your spine, bringing energy and a feeling of effortlessness to your daily activities like dressing yourself or fun activities such as playing tennis and golf.

**You should be feeling the work** in your shoulder blades, chest, spine, ribs, and obliques.

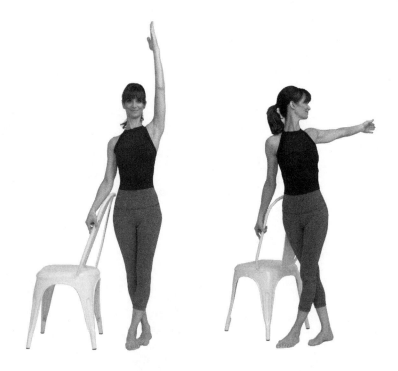

1. Stand next to the back of your chair, holding it with your right hand.

2. Raise your left arm above your head.

3. Place your left foot directly in front of your right foot, making sure that the soles of your feet are flat on the ground and not rolling in or out at your ankles. You may have to adjust the placement of your feet in order to make sure that they are flat on the ground.

4. Pull your left arm toward the back of the room, sweeping in a circular motion and finishing with your arm at shoulder height.

5. Pull the arm to the back of the room and continue the corkscrew motion as you twist further.

6. This should take 10 seconds.

7. Raise your left arm above your head and place your feet together as you face the front. Bend your knees.

8. Slowly bend toward the chair, lengthening the side of your body to get a deep stretch through the outside of your torso. Use the arm to deepen the stretch by pulling it out of the socket toward the wall.

9. Return to the starting position with the left leg crossed over the right.

10. Repeat the complete sequence 3 times before changing sides.

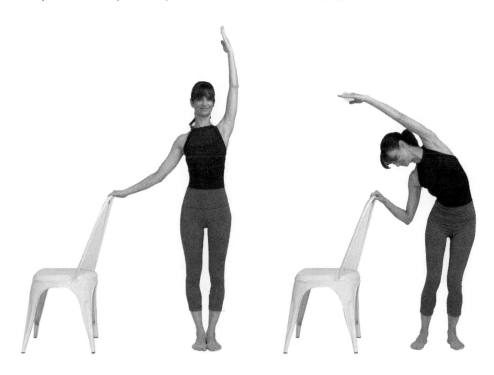

# SPINE STRETCHES

**Use visualization to stimulate your neurons:** Imagine that you are a cat slowly massaging your spine, as you move side-to-side.

**This sequence will** relieve tension throughout the muscles and connective tissue of your back, from your shoulders into your hips. This will take all the tension out of your body at the end of this workout. Do this feel-good exercise at any time of day if you feel tension in your back.

**You should be feeling the work** in your spine, shoulder blades, and glutes.

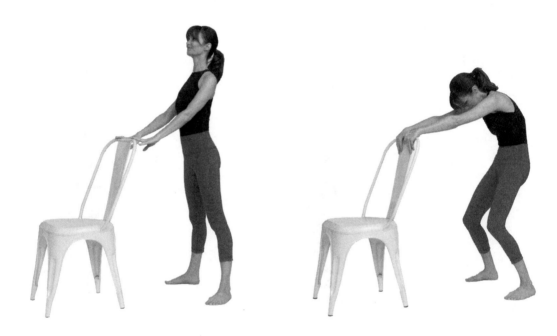

1. Stand facing the back of your chair, holding the chair with both hands.
2. Place your feet wider than hip-width distance apart and bend your knees.
3. Round your back, lift your shoulders, and tuck your tailbone under as much as possible.
4. Shift your weight gently side to side to release tension on both sides of the spine. This relaxed mini side-to-side shifting should take 10 seconds. This should feel really good. It

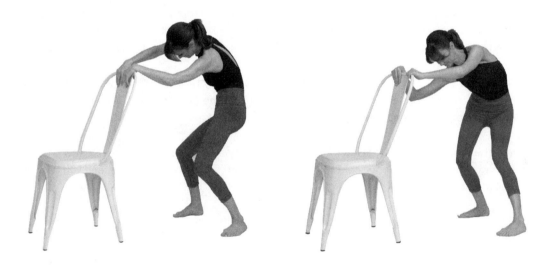

shouldn't hurt. Move the way a cat does when it stretches its spine. Allow your spine to articulate throughout the exercise, don't hold it straight.

5. Repeat 8 times before returning to your starting position with your back and knees completely straight.

6. Take a deep breath, inhaling and exhaling slowly, and repeat a second time.

## PART TWO OF WORKOUT 2: **Floor Exercises (Optional)**

ABDOMINALS

The next two exercises are sit-ups to engage your abdominal muscles. Remember:

- When doing sit-ups, do not press the center of your spine into the floor, as is traditionally taught. Pressing it into the floor actually damages the spine and can lead to slipped and bulging discs.

- Use this trick to help you identify the muscles to engage in a sit-up: lie on your back with your knees bent. Put your hands between your pubic bone and your hipbones and cough. When you cough, you will feel your transverse abdominis muscles contract. Those are the ones we want to engage as they are crucial in strengthening and flattening your stomach.

- When you lift your shoulders off of the floor, imagine that you are pulling your pubic bone and your ribs toward each other. Never do a sit-up by leading with your head and using the head and neck to pull the upper body off the floor. This will cause neck damage and headaches and will do little to strengthen your stomach.

- As you do your sit-up, move very slowly so that you only have your muscles to lift you off the floor. Do not use momentum or speed to lift off the floor rapidly. Slow movement is more effective in strengthening your muscles.

- Your head will naturally be lifted off the floor as your shoulders rise up. Because you are not pulling with your head, your chin will not drop toward your chest and your face will remain looking at the ceiling.

- By keeping your head aligned with your spine during the sit-ups, you will protect your neck from injury.

# SIMPLE SIT-UPS

This sequence will strengthen your abdominal muscles, increasing support to your back and improving your posture.

You should be feeling the work in your rectus abdominis, transverse abdominis, obliques, and psoas.

> If you have a rounded back that prevents you from maintaining clean alignment when lying on the floor, place a firm cushion under your head. This will straighten the spine and avoid compression in your neck.

1. Lie flat on the ground, knees bent, feet placed flat on the ground, hip-width distance apart.

2. Place your hands behind your ears, fingers barely touching your head while opening your elbows as wide as possible.

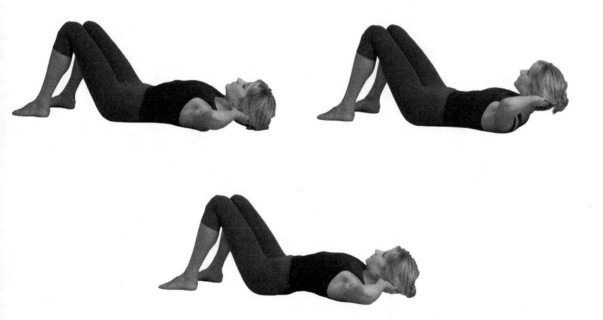

3. Following the notes on page 274 on abdominal exercises, contract your abs to raise your upper back, counting to 3 to raise and 3 to lower.

4. Exhale when you contract your abs to lift the shoulders, and inhale as you lower them.

5. Maintain control of your stomach muscles the entire time, making sure not to relax them or grip them in extreme tension.

6. Repeat 16 to 32 times.

# ELBOW-TO-KNEE SIT-UPS

**This sequence will** strengthen your abdominal muscles, increase support to your back, and improve your posture.

**You should be feeling the work** in your rectus abdominis, transverse abdominis, obliques, and psoas.

> If you have a rounded back that prevents you from maintaining clean alignment when lying on the floor, place a firm cushion under your head. This will straighten the spine and avoid compression in your neck.

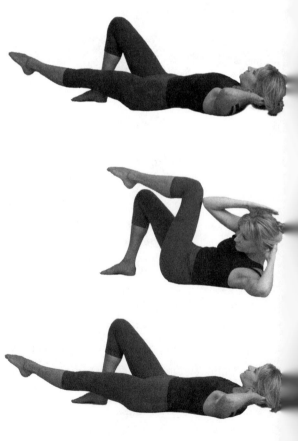

1. Lie flat on the ground, knees bent, right foot placed flat on the ground, and your left leg extended with your toes pointed, 3 inches off the ground.

2. Place your hands behind your ears, fingers barely touching your head while opening your elbows as wide as possible.

3. Following the notes on abdominal exercises on page 274, contract your abs to raise your upper back as you twist your torso, bringing your right shoulder toward your left knee, counting 3 to raise and 3 to lower.

4. Exhale when you contract your abs to lift the shoulders, and inhale as you lower them.

5. Maintain control of your stomach muscles the entire time, making sure not to relax them or grip them in extreme tension.

6. Repeat 8 times per leg.

7. Repeat this entire sequence twice.

LEGS

# SIDE LEG LIFTS

**Use visualization to stimulate your neurons:** Imagine pulling your leg away from the hip socket during the entire exercise and that you are being pulled from the tip of your head in one direction and the tips of your toes in the other, elongating every muscle and joint in your body.

**This sequence will** strengthen your hips while slenderizing and toning your legs and glutes. It will hydrate and reinforce the crimp in the ligaments of the hips and knees, giving you strength and balance.

**You should be feeling the work** in your hips and throughout your back (if you are correctly lengthening your muscles throughout the exercise).

> Make side leg lifts more comfortable by placing your hip in the hole of a firm hemorrhoid cushion (not the inflatable kind).

1. Lay on your left side, with your left knee bent and your right leg extended with pointed toes touching the floor.
2. Bend your left arm, laying the forearm directly under your shoulder so that it acts as a support for your torso.
3. Important: place your right arm in front for additional support.

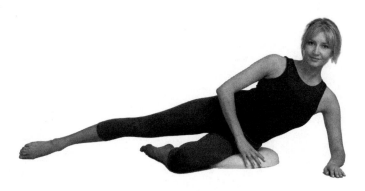

4. Slide your right foot along the floor, away from the body, lifting it when you can't slide any further. This makes the leg feel very heavy; however, this will strengthen and slenderize your legs.

5. Take 3 seconds to lift the leg and 3 seconds to lower it.

6. Repeat 8 times with a pointed foot, and 8 times with a flexed foot.

7. Repeat this sequence again.

8. Shake out your hips and change sides.

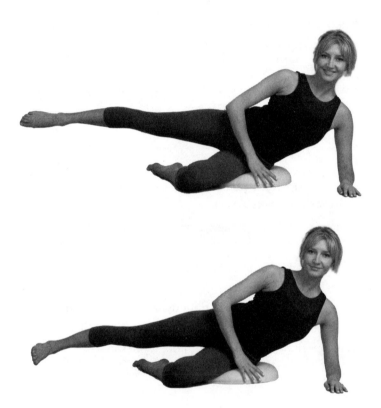

DEEP STRETCHES

# SEATED HIP STRETCH

This sequence will loosen congealed connective tissue in your hips, glutes, and lower back, which will relieve pain and improve mobility. It will stretch the muscles of your glutes right through the full erector spinae muscles to improve your posture.

You should be feeling the work in your spine and hips.

> If you have tight hamstrings or back muscles, sit on a riser.

1. Sit on the floor, with your left leg extended and toes pointed and your right leg bent. If you can't keep your left leg straight, bend your knee.

2. Cross your right foot over your left leg, keeping the foot flat on the floor. If you can't cross your foot over, keep it beside your leg.

3. Embrace your right knee with your left arm as you twist your spine toward the back of the room. Place the right hand on the floor behind your back to help you pull your spine upward.

4. Pull your right knee toward your chest with your left arm. You will feel a deep stretch in the hips.

5. Count to 6 and release the stretch.

6. Repeat 3 times before changing legs.

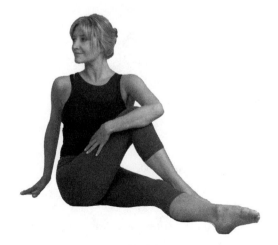

# SEATED WINDMILL

**Use visualization to stimulate your neurons:** Imagine that your arms are the blades of a giant windmill. As one blade moves upward, the opposite blade will mirror the movement downward as if they are making a giant circle. As you are moving the arms in a giant circle, imagine you are pulling them away from the shoulder socket to maximize the lengthening of the spine.

**This sequence will** work the large sheets of fascia in your torso, spine, hips, and upper legs.

**You should be feeling the work** in your back, chest, pectorals, calves, hamstrings, and IT bands.

> If you have tight hamstrings or back muscles, sit on a riser.

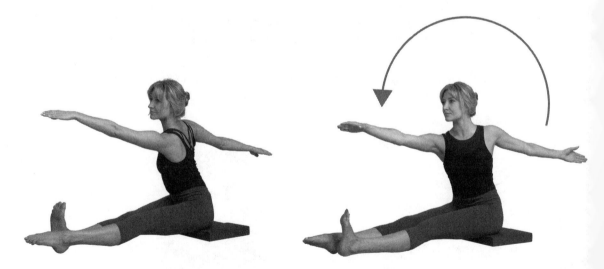

1. Sit on the floor with both legs extended. If your hamstrings are tight, you may not be able to straighten your knees. Do not worry. This exercise will still stretch your hamstrings.

2. Point your left foot and flex your right foot.

3. Extend your left arm over your left leg and reach behind you with your right arm, while twisting your torso.

4. Keep your back completely straight, do not round your back.

5. Keep your shoulders down, while imagining that you are slipping your shoulder blades into your back pocket.

6. Bend forward as much as you can without rounding your back or bending your knees.

7. Start the windmill, raising your right arm over your head, pulling it as far away from your shoulders as you can, while doing the opposite motion with your left arm.

8. As you move your arms, switch the position of your feet, from pointed to flexed or flexed to pointed.

9. Each half-windmill should take 10 seconds.

10. Repeat 8 times.

# SEATED IT BAND STRETCH

**This sequence will** stretch the IT band, a wide strip of connective tissue that runs down the length of the outer thigh, from the top of the pelvis to the shin. When it becomes tight, it causes arthritis in the knee, chronic knee pain, and possibly the need for knee replacement.

**You should be feeling the work** in the outside of your thighs. You may feel a minor discomfort near your knee. As long as it is not a sharp pain, do not worry.

> If you have tight hamstrings or back muscles, sit on a riser.

1. Sit on the floor with both legs extended. If your hamstrings are tight, you may not be able to straighten your knees. Do not worry. This exercise will still stretch your hamstrings.
2. Point your right foot and flex your left foot.
3. Place your right hand across your left leg while simultaneously twisting your spine in the same direction.
4. Place your left hand on the floor behind you, using it to help keep your spine straight. Do not round your spine during this exercise.
5. With the fingers of your right arm, walk down the outside your left leg as far as you can, keeping your back straight and your left foot as flexed as possible.
6. Hold for 6 seconds.
7. Return to your starting position and relax your leg.
8. Repeat 4 times on each leg.

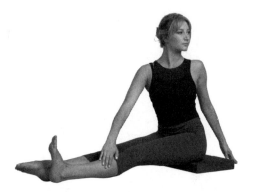 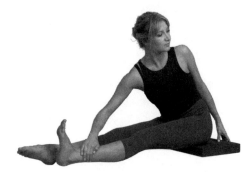

# ROW A BOAT WITH FLEXED FEET

**Use visualization to stimulate your neurons:** Imagine rowing a boat with both arms and then lifting weights above your head.

This sequence will work the large sheets of fascia in your torso, spine, hips, and legs.

You should be feeling the work in your back, chest, pectorals, calves, and hamstrings.

> If you have tight hamstrings or back muscles, sit on a riser.

1. Sit on the floor with both legs extended. Slightly bend your knees.

2. Flex your feet and pull your spine upward.

3. Raise your arms with bent elbows, lifting upward. The palms of your hands should be facing the front.

4. Imagine you are pushing a weight toward your feet, keeping your back straight as you bend forward. This should take 6 seconds.

5. When you reach your maximum ability to keep your back straight, round your back. Relax with your back rounded and wiggle around for an additional 6 seconds.

6. Round your back and grab the imaginary oars of a rowboat.

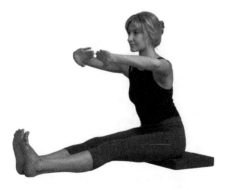 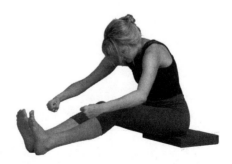

7. Pull the oars back with resistance as though you were really rowing a boat. This should take 6 seconds.

8. When you arrive with your arms close to your ears, do a giant shoulder joint rotation, finishing with your hands beside your shoulders.

9. Extend your arms above your head.

10. Once your elbows have straightened completely, relax your shoulders and pull your arms, spine, and torso, with full strength, toward the ceiling. This should take 6 seconds.

11. Repeat this full sequence 4 times.

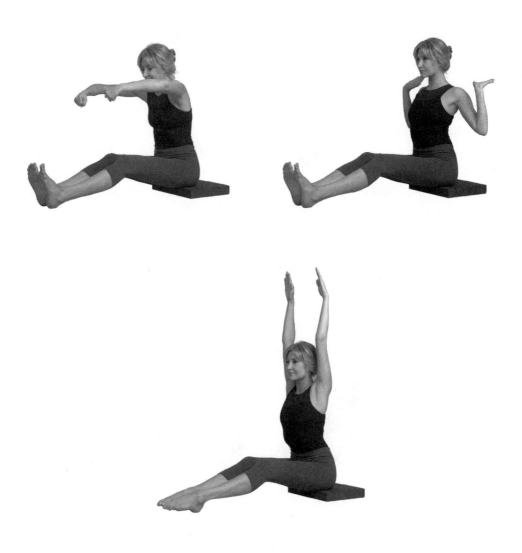

# WORKOUT 3, DAYS 21–30

### PART ONE OF WORKOUT 3: Standing and Chair Exercises

### PART TWO OF WORKOUT 3: Floor Exercises (Optional)

**PART ONE OF WORKOUT 3: Standing and Chair Exercises**

## STANDING EXERCISES

**WARM-UP SEQUENCE**

The warm-up involves five different exercises, each of which should be repeated 16 times. When you finish all five, start again from the beginning. Repeat at least twice. Warming up should last a minimum of 3 minutes. These zero-impact cardiovascular exercises will raise your body temperature by warming up your muscles and releasing tension throughout your full body.

Be sure to maintain a steady deep-breathing pattern throughout your warm-up.

# SINGLE-ARM HALF-CIRCLE SWINGS

**Use visualization to stimulate your neurons:** Imagine swinging your arm like a pendulum.

This sequence will increase blood circulation in your full body to warm up the musculature.

You should be feeling the work in your thighs, ankles, shoulders, and spine.

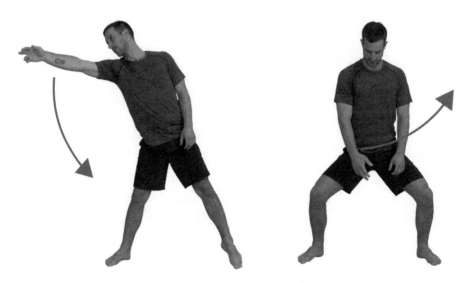

1. Stand in a wide plié stance. The degree of safe turnout varies from person to person. With the correct foot placement, you shouldn't feel any stress in your hips, knees, or feet. Adjust your feet accordingly and choose the degree of turnout that works best for you.

2. Shift your weight onto your right leg and point your left foot.

3. Lift your right arm, bending sideways to the right. Keep your left arm relaxed and by your side.

4. Lower your arm, bending your knees as your arm reaches center.

5. Shift your weight to your left foot and bend sideways, straightening both legs, pointing the right foot, and raising your arm to the opposite side. Imagine your right arm is a pendulum swinging easily within the shoulder joint.

6. When you bend sideways, focus on letting each vertebra bend so that your spine does not stay rigid.

7. Keep your legs, arms, and spine relaxed throughout the arm swings.

8. Repeat 4 times before changing arms.

9. Repeat the sequence with each arm.

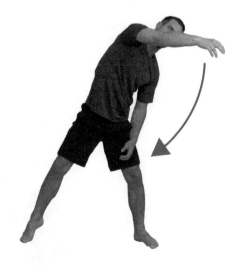

# SINGLE-ARM FULL ROTATION

**Use visualization to stimulate your neurons:** Imagine drawing a large circle with one arm.

**This sequence will** increase blood circulation in your full body to warm up the musculature.

**You should be feeling the work** in your thighs, ankles, shoulders, and spine.

1. Stand in a wide plié stance. The degree of safe turnout varies from person to person. With the correct foot placement, you shouldn't feel any stress in your hips, knees, or feet. Adjust your feet accordingly and choose the degree of turnout that works best for you.

2. Shift your weight onto your left leg and point your right foot.

3. Lift your left arm, bending sideways to the left. Keep your right arm relaxed and by your side.

4. Lower your arm, bending your knees as your arms reach center.

5. Shift your weight to your right foot and bend sideways, straightening both legs, pointing the left foot, and raising your left arm to the opposite side, over your head, and back to the starting position. Imagine your left arm is a pendulum swinging easily within the shoulder joint.

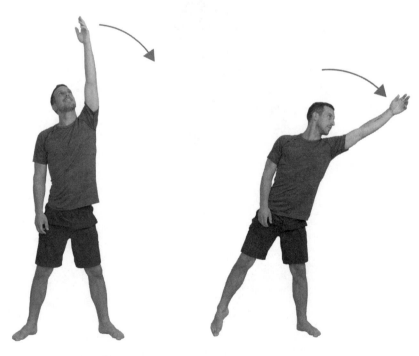

6. When you bend sideways, focus on letting each vertebra bend so that your spine does not stay rigid.

7. Keep your legs, arms, and spine relaxed throughout the arm swings.

8. Repeat 4 times in each direction before changing arms.

9. Repeat the complete sequence.

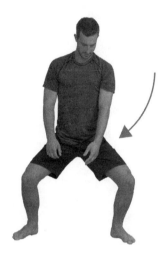
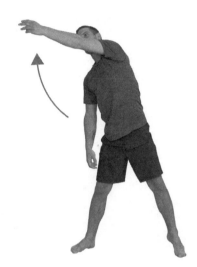

# DOUBLE-ARM HALF-CIRCLE SWING

**Use visualization to stimulate your neurons:** Imagine your arms are the pendulum on a clock, swinging freely. Your legs, while moving up and down, are acting like an old-fashioned water pump. Visualize this action pumping your blood throughout your body, increasing your circulation. This is how the cardiovascular system is designed to work; skeletal muscles are designed to be a partner to the cardiac muscle in the distribution of blood throughout your body.

This sequence will increase blood circulation in your full body to warm up the musculature and connective tissue.

You should be feeling the work in your thighs, ankles, shoulders, and spine.

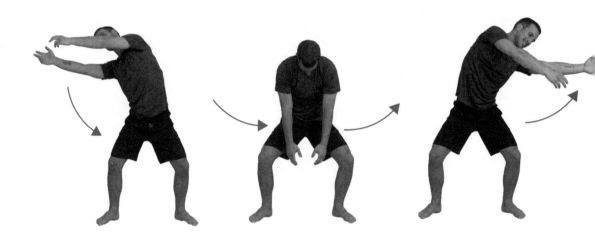

1. Stand in a wide plié stance. The degree of safe turnout varies from person to person. With the correct foot placement, you shouldn't feel any stress in your hips, knees, or feet. Adjust your feet accordingly and choose the degree of turnout that works best for you.

2. Raise both arms to the right and lean, bending your spine toward the right.

3. Move your arms toward the floor and up to the opposite side, imagining both arms are a pendulum swinging easily within the shoulder joints.

4. While shifting from side to side, pump the knees up and down gently to warm up the thighs.

5. When you bend sideways, focus on letting each vertebra bend so that your spine does not stay rigid.

6. Keep your legs, arms, and spine relaxed throughout the arm swings.

7. Repeat 4 times in each direction.

8. Repeat the complete sequence.

# DOUBLE-ARM FULL ROTATION

**Use visualization to stimulate your neurons:** Imagine drawing a large circle with your arms.

This sequence will increase blood circulation in your full body to warm up the musculature and connective tissue.

**You should be feeling the work** in your thighs, ankles, shoulders, and spine.

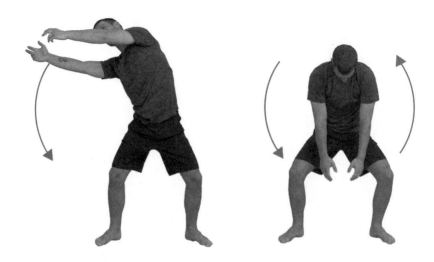

1. Stand in a wide plié stance. The degree of safe turnout varies from person to person. With the correct foot placement, you shouldn't feel any stress in your hips, knees, or feet. Adjust your feet accordingly and choose the degree of turnout that works best for you.

2. Raise both arms to the right and lean, bending your spine toward the right.

3. Move your arms toward the floor and up to the opposite side, overhead, and back to the starting position, imagining both arms are a pendulum swinging easily within the shoulder joints.

4. While shifting from side to side, pump the knees up and down gently to warm up the thighs.

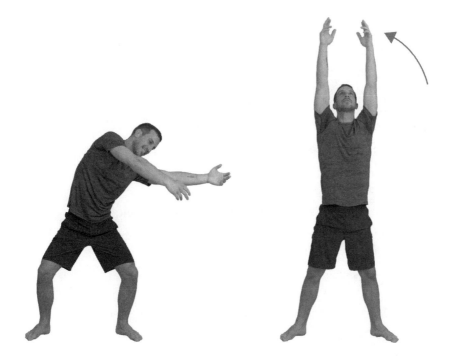

5. When you bend sideways, focus on letting each vertebra bend so that your spine does not stay rigid.

6. Keep your legs, arms, and spine relaxed throughout the arm swings.

7. Repeat 4 times in each direction.

8. Repeat the complete sequence.

# DIAGONAL TWISTS

Please note that this stretch is the same as the one you did in Workout 2.

**Use visualization to stimulate your neurons:** Imagine twisting around your spine as though it is a corkscrew.

**This sequence will** warm up all of the muscles of your spine while loosening congealed connective tissue. It will also improve posture and prevent back pain.

**You should be feeling the work** in your spine, shoulders, hips, and knees.

1. Stand with your feet slightly wider than hip-width distance apart. Bend your knees and elbows while bringing your hands to touch your collarbones.

2. Shift onto the left leg, raise the right arm in front of you diagonally and the left arm diagonally behind as you twist on your spine.

3. Point the right foot behind you.

4. Return to the transition position, both knees and elbows bent.

5. Repeat this diagonal twist in the other direction. These side-to-side shifts should be very smooth and fluid.

6. Repeat 8 times on each side.

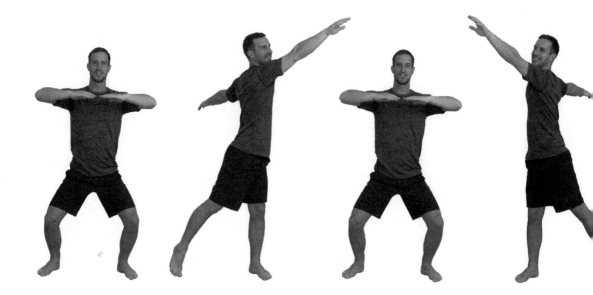

TRADEMARK SEQUENCE

# SPINAL ROLL

**Use visualization to stimulate your neurons:** Picture your spine as a bicycle chain, rolling up one link at a time, starting at the base and finishing at the top.

**This sequence will** prevent and reverse back pain while improving your posture by loosening and hydrating the sheets of connective tissue in your entire back. It will also stretch and strengthen all of the muscles and ligaments that support the spine.

**You should be feeling the work** in your spine, shoulders, and hips.

1. Stand with your feet parallel and comfortably placed on the floor, slightly wider than hip-width distance apart. Do not force your feet to turn in or out.

2. Place your hands on your knees as you bend them.

3. Round your spine, making sure that your lower back is as tucked under as possible and that your shoulders do not drop beyond your knees. Do not stick your bum out or arch your back, as this will compress your spine rather than stretch it.

**Side View**

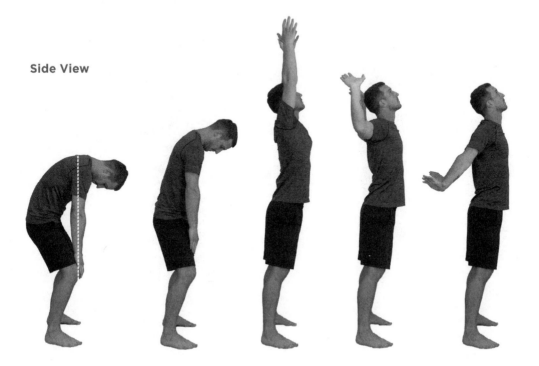

**Front View**

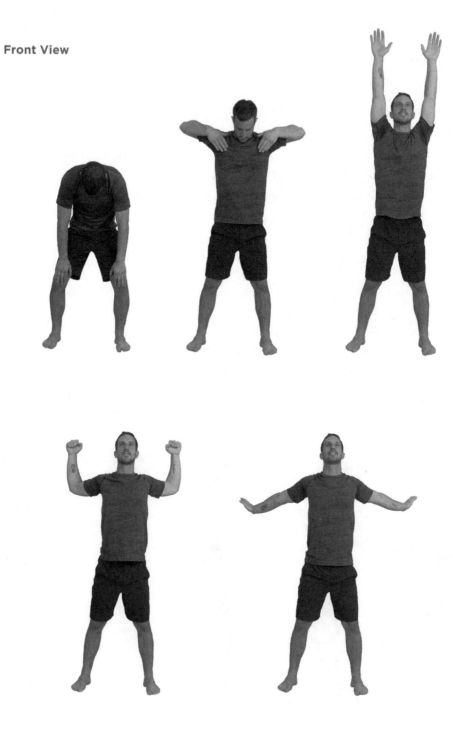

4. Start the spinal roll from the lowest vertebra in your spine and slowly roll up one vertebra at a time, trying to feel each vertebra as it shifts into an elongated spinal position.

5. As you are rolling up, follow your body with your hands until you reach your shoulders.

6. Simultaneously straighten the knees as your arms reach shoulder height.

7. Extend the arms above your head, raising your hands toward the ceiling while relaxing the shoulder sockets. Do not tense your muscles. By relaxing your shoulders, you will be able to raise your arms higher above your head. Count 6 seconds as you are extending the arms above your head.

8. Make a fist, bend the elbows, and relax your shoulders. Imagine you are dropping your shoulder blades in a back pocket, all the while not letting your back arch.

9. Trying to relax your pectoral muscles, pull the bent elbows behind your shoulders as much as possible. Once again, don't let your back move. By locking your spine in an elongated position without arching it, you are stretching the chest and pectoral muscles, which will improve your posture, and training the spine to decompress by pulling up and not sinking down.

10. Open your hands as much as possible while straightening your elbows. Hold that position for another 6 seconds as you pull your arms farther back.

11. Repeat the complete sequence 3 times. Each sequence should take at least 20 seconds.

12. Move slowly the entire time. Don't stop and start or make jerky movements. Keep the movements flowing.

# SHOULDER BLAST

**Use visualization to stimulate your neurons:** Imagine your shoulder blades slipping and sliding as they rotate up and down throughout this exercise.

**This sequence will** prevent back and shoulder pain as well as improve your posture. It will also open your chest and improve your ability to breathe and stand up straight. In addition to working on your shoulder blades, it will work directly on your shoulder joints. By twisting your arms within the joints as well as moving the arms in a circle from back to front, you will clean out congealed connective tissue in the joint itself and realign by stretching and strengthening all of the attaching ligaments, tendons, and muscles of the shoulder joint. This will liberate your shoulders and will restore the full range of motion into the arms. When your arm has a limited range of motion, you'll feel the effect throughout your body.

**You should be feeling the work** in your spine, shoulders, and shoulder blades.

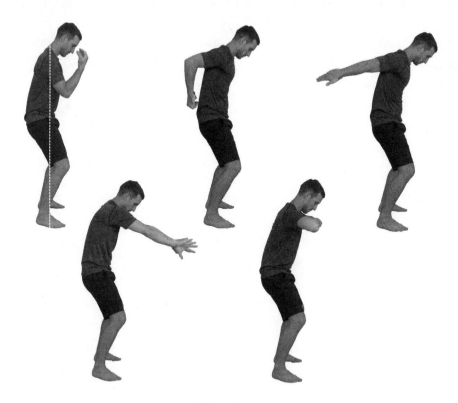

**Side View**

1. Stand with your feet parallel and comfortably placed on the floor, slightly wider than hip-width distance. Do not force your feet to turn in or out.

2. Place your spine in Neutral C, shoulders down (see page 111).

3. Bend your elbows, pulling the palms of your hands toward your shoulders.

4. Pull your elbows behind you, keeping them bent and as close together as possible. This will force your shoulders to rise up, which is correct.

5. When you can't lift your elbows any higher behind you, straighten them.

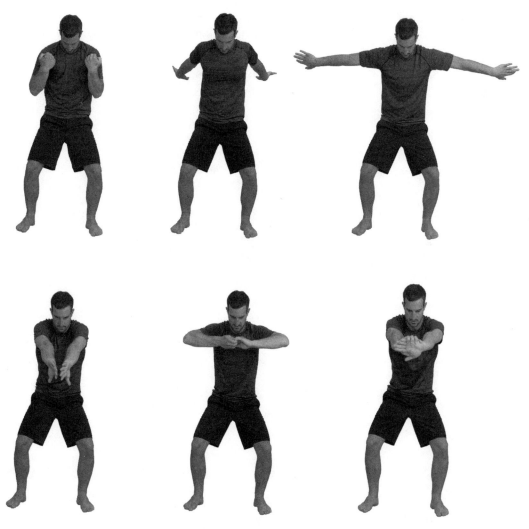

**Front View**

6. You should be feeling this stretch in the entire shoulder joint.

7. Rotate your arms within the shoulder joint. Take your time to do this.

8. As slowly as possible, bring your arms in front of your body, circling from back to front and keeping them at shoulder height throughout the rotation.

9. Once you arrive in front of your shoulders, grab your fingers and pull your hands to your chest while keeping your elbows at shoulder height.

10. Make sure your fingers stay locked together while you are trying to separate your hands. Lift your shoulders as high as possible while doing this. You will feel a lot of tension in your shoulder blades.

11. Relax the tension in your fingers. Keep your hands together while pressing them toward the front of the room, maintaining shoulder height. You should feel a liberation in your shoulder blades.

12. The whole sequence should take you about 20 seconds.

13. Repeat 4 times.

# WINDMILLS

**Use visualization to stimulate your neurons:** Imagine that your arms are the blades of a giant windmill. As one blade moves upward, the opposite blade will mirror the movement downward in the opposite direction, as if you are moving the arms in a giant circle. Visualize pulling your arms out of their sockets to maximize the lengthening of the spine.

**This sequence will** rebalance your spine by stretching and strengthening the surrounding muscles and connective tissue while working the full body. It will relieve back pain and improve your posture.

**You should be feeling the work** in your spine and shoulders, and from your glutes down your legs and into your calves.

1. Stand with your feet wide apart and both legs straight. Place your right leg in front and your left leg behind.
2. Raise your left arm above your head and place your right arm beside your hips.
3. Lower your left arm in front and raise the right arm behind in a windmill motion as you bend your right knee and lean forward, twisting your spine at the same time as your arms move. Keep the arms moving simultaneously, and don't let one move without the other.
4. Count 15 seconds to draw this half windmill.
5. Reverse the movements to return to the starting position. You have completed a full windmill.
6. Repeat for a total of 2 full windmills before changing sides. Repeat the same sequence on the other side.
7. Repeat both sides again.

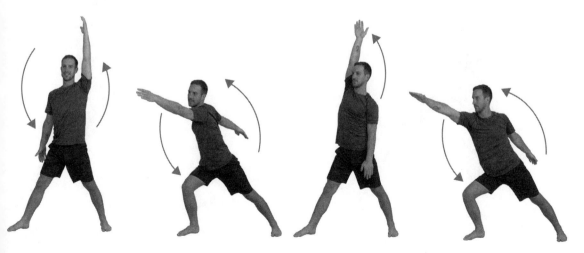

# WINDMILLS WITH RELAXING AND RELEASING

**Use visualization to stimulate your neurons:** Imagine building up tension in your muscles before deeply releasing and relaxing them. This technique safely and effortlessly releases tension in your muscles to increase your flexibility in a short amount of time.

**This sequence will** rebalance your spine by stretching and strengthening the surrounding muscles while working the full body. It will relieve back pain and improve your posture.

**You should be feeling the work** in your spine and shoulders, and from your glutes down your legs and into your calves.

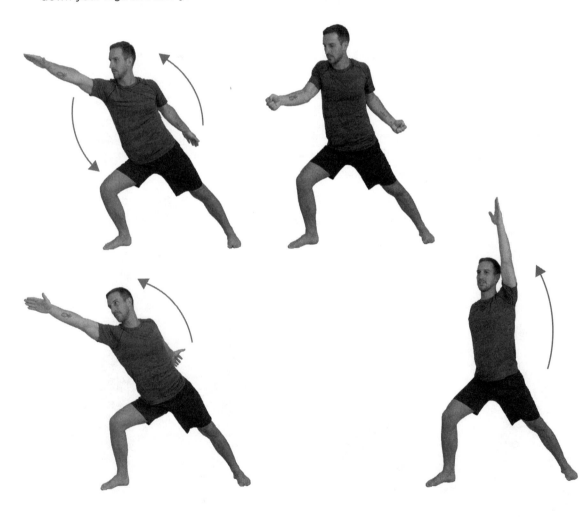

1. Stand in a front lunge, with your right leg forward and bent and your left leg back and extended.

2. Extend your right arm over your right knee, slightly above shoulder height, and your left arm over your left leg, slightly below shoulder height.

3. Keep your hips facing the right knee while you twist your spine toward your left leg.

4. Contract your fists, arms, and shoulders as much as possible, holding the contraction for about 3 seconds.

5. Take a few seconds to relax the contraction.

6. Imagine that your arms are being pulled away from each other, stretching them away from the sockets as much as possible. Let your spine twist as much as possible as your arms are stretching out. You will notice that your spine can twist farther than before.

7. Change the arms by doing a windmill (see page 301). Your left arm should now be in front and your right arm in back.

8. Repeat the contraction and the relaxation on this side, followed by the stretching twist of the spine.

9. This entire sequence, from right arm to left arm, should take about 30 seconds.

10. Repeat 2 times on the same leg before changing legs.

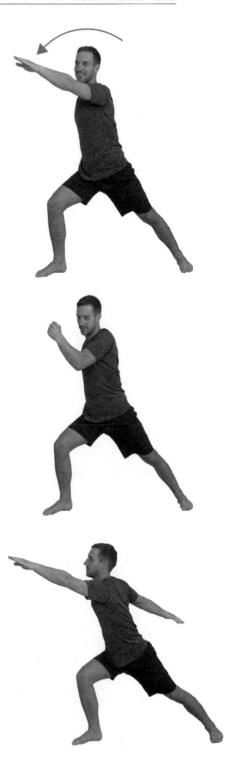

ARMS

# TRICEPS AND DELTOID ARM SEQUENCE

**Use visualization to stimulate your neurons:** Imagine standing with your arms extended fully out to your sides; a person is on either side of you, pulling your arms away from you. Picture slipping your shoulders into your back pocket throughout this entire exercise. Don't let your shoulders lift up and down at any time during this sequence. As you are pumping the arms up and down, imagine that you are fighting against an invisible resistance that is preventing you from moving your arms more than 6 inches in either direction.

**This sequence will** stretch compressed deltoid muscles (your shoulder muscles), releasing tension in the shoulder joints. It will realign the connective tissue of your shoulder joints, which is the fascia around your muscles as well as the ligaments that attach your arms to your shoulders. It will increase the strength and mobility of your shoulders while relieving pain and healing injuries. This sequence will also improve your posture and stress the bones of your shoulders and spine to avoid or reverse osteoporosis.

**You should be feeling the work** in your shoulders, chest, and underarms.

1. Stand with your feet parallel and comfortably placed on the floor, slightly wider than hip-width distance apart. Do not force your feet to turn in or out.

2. Your knees should be slightly bent and your spine completely straight throughout the entire exercise.

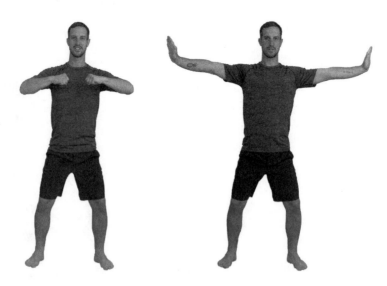

3. Bend your elbows and lift them to shoulder height. Rest your hands on your chest.

4. Extend your arms at shoulder height, keeping the elbows straight (if you can).

5. Flex your wrists upward, straightening the fingers as much as possible.

6. Pump your arms downward, about 6 inches, fighting against an invisible resistance, for a count of 2.

7. Release the tension in your underarm and return to the starting position.

8. Repeat 8 times before returning to the beginning arm position with your arms extended at shoulder height.

9. Repeat this sequence of 8 pumps downward, 4 times (total of 32 pumps).

10. Modify this sequence by pumping toward the back of the room. Lock the spine in an erect posture to avoid arching your back and don't push your arms farther than 3 inches from the starting position.

11. Repeat for a total of 8 pumps before returning to the beginning arm position, with your elbows bent and hands resting on your chest.

12. Repeat this sequence of 8 pumps backward, 4 times (total of 32 pumps).

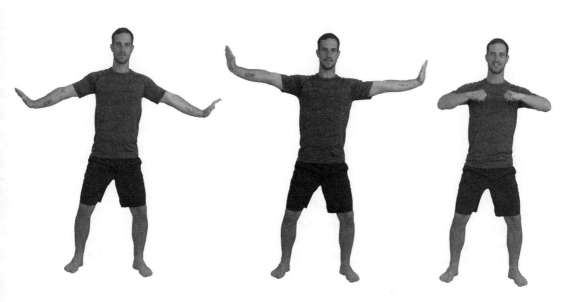

PLIÉS

# PLIÉS WITH CEILING REACHES

**Use visualization to stimulate your neurons:** Imagine doing your pliés (knee bends) between two glass walls. This image will stop you from bending forward and sticking out your bum. If you have a little turnout in your hips that prevents you from pointing your toes outward, don't force your feet. Place them in their natural turnout, which might be limited. This will force you to slightly bend your back forward to maintain your balance.

**This sequence will** stretch and strengthen your quads, glutes, and back muscles. It will relieve knee pain by elongating the quadriceps, therefore decompressing the knee joint. It will hydrate and loosen the sheets of fascia that surround your thighs, glutes, and lower back. This exercise will realign the connective tissue fibers, helping to maintain the rebound action in your hips and knees. This is a powerful exercise for people with knee pain, arthritis, and unresolved injuries.

**You should be feeling the work** in your quadriceps, hips, ribs, and arms.

> If you suffer from chronic knee pain, bend your knees only as far as you are capable of before triggering the pain message. To heal knee pain, you must bend your knees, but it's important that you not go into the pain mode. You should find that your pain disappears quite rapidly when you are bending your knees just enough but not too much.

1. Place your feet wider than hip-width distance apart, in a comfortable turnout that starts at your hips. Your turnout starts with the rotation of the hips, not with the placement of your feet. Once you find your maximum safe hip turnout, make sure you are standing correctly on the full soles of your feet. Standing on the soles of your feet will automatically protect your knees from twisting.

2. Keep a straight spine and imagine that you are pulling it toward the ceiling, lengthening it during this entire exercise. Do not relax this pulling-up effort on your muscles; keep working hard to lengthen them throughout the entire exercise. You will see a huge change in your posture from working in this mode.

3. Bend your knees as deeply as possible, stopping the moment you feel any twinge of pain. Do not let the knees extend beyond your toes. You might have to widen your stance in order to keep this from happening. It is very good for your inner hip flexibility to keep a wide stance.

4. Raise your arms to your sides, with your elbows completely bent, and make fists with your hands.

5. Lift your left arm up, trying to touch the ceiling, relaxing the shoulder to permit the arm to rise as high as you possibly can.

6. Once you reach as high as you can, relax your ribs and shoulder joint and reach farther (you will be able to).

7. When your arm has extended up as far as it can, spread your fingers as wide as possible.

8. This ceiling reach sequence should take 10 seconds from start to finish.

9. Return to the starting position.

10. Alternating sides, repeat 8 times.

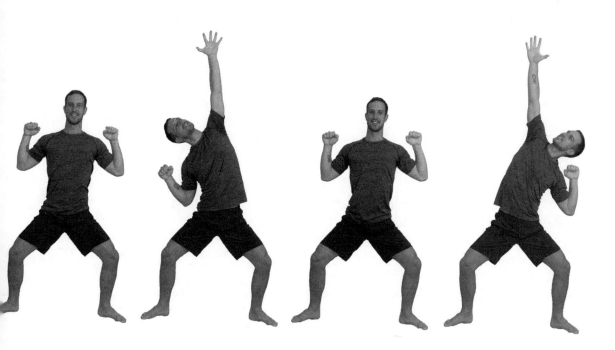

# PLIÉS WITH DEEP SIDE BENDS

**Use visualization to stimulate your neurons:** Using the same imagery on the placement of your feet as in the previous exercise (hint: two glass walls), imagine that as you bend sideways, you are squeezed between two glass walls to prevent you from rounding your back or sticking your bum out. Visualize creating more space between each of your thirty-three individual vertebra as you bend sideways.

**This sequence will** improve your posture, lengthen your spine, and stress the entire skeleton of your body to help reverse osteoporosis, in addition to everything described in the first plié sequence.

**You should be feeling the work** in your quadriceps, hips, ribs, obliques, back, and arms. This is a full-body deep stretching and strengthening exercise.

> If you suffer from chronic knee pain, bend your knees only as far as you are capable of before triggering the pain message. To heal knee pain, you must bend your knees, but it's important that you not go into the pain mode. You should find that your pain disappears quite rapidly when you are bending your knees just enough but not too much.

1. Place your feet wider than hip-width distance apart, in a comfortable turnout that starts at your hips. Your turnout starts with the rotation of the hips, not with the placement of your feet. Once you find your safe maximum hip turnout, make sure you are standing correctly on the full soles of your feet. Standing on the soles of your feet will automatically protect your knees from twisting.

2. Keep your spine straight and imagine that you are pulling it toward the ceiling, lengthening it during this entire exercise. Do not relax this pulling-up effort on your muscles; keep working hard to lengthen them throughout the entire exercise. You will see a huge change in your posture from working in this mode.

3. Bend your knees as deeply as possible, stopping the moment you feel any twinge of pain. Do not let the knees extend beyond your toes. You might have to widen your stance in order to accomplish this. It is very good for your inner hip flexibility to keep a wide stance.

4. Raise your arms to your sides, with your elbows completely bent, and make fists with your hands.

5. Lift your right arm up beside your ear as you bend as far to the left as possible.

6. This should take 5 seconds to bend sideways and 5 seconds to return to the starting position.

7. Repeat on the other side.

8. Alternating sides, repeat 8 times.

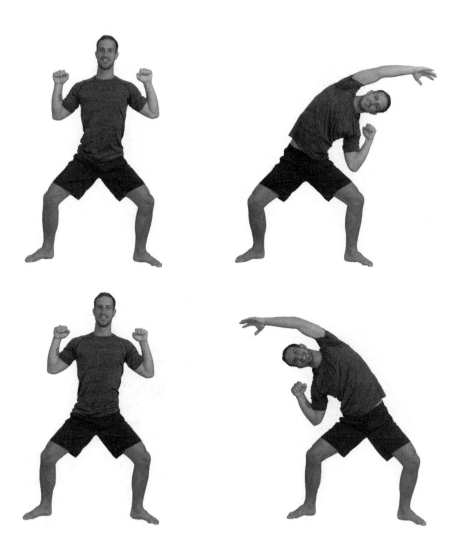

# PLIÉS WITH DEEP SIDE LUNGES

**Use visualization to stimulate your neurons:** Use the same imagery on the placement of your feet as in the previous exercises.

This sequence will improve your posture, lengthen your spine, and stress the entire skeleton of your body to help reverse osteoporosis, in addition to everything described in the first plié sequence.

You should be feeling the work in your quadriceps, hips, ribs, obliques, back, and arms. This is a full-body deep stretching and strengthening exercise.

If you suffer from chronic knee pain, bend your knees only as far as you are capable of before triggering the pain message. To heal knee pain, you must bend your knees, but it's important that you not go into the pain mode. You should find that your pain disappears quite rapidly when you are bending your knees just enough but not too much.

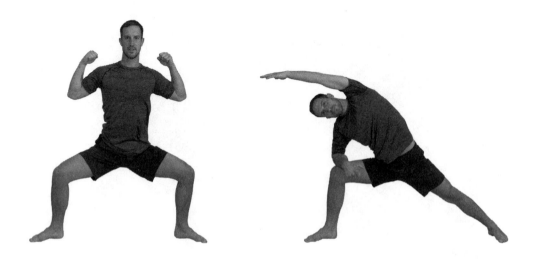

1. Place your feet wider than hip-width distance apart, in a comfortable turnout that starts at your hips. Your turnout starts with the rotation of the hips, not with the placement of your feet. Once you find your maximum safe hip turnout, make sure you are standing correctly on the full soles of your feet. Standing on the soles of your feet will automatically protect your knees from twisting.

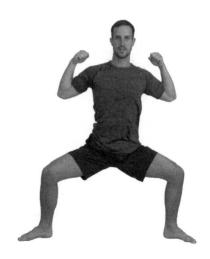

2. Keep your spine straight and imagine that you are pulling it toward the ceiling, lengthening it during this entire exercise. Do not relax this pulling-up effort on your muscles; keep working hard to lengthen them throughout the entire exercise. You will see a huge change in your posture from working in this mode.

3. Bend your knees as deeply as possible, stopping the moment you feel any twinge of pain. Do not let the knees extend beyond your toes. You might have to widen your stance in order to keep this from happening. It is very good for your inner hip flexibility to use a wide stance.

4. Raise your arms to your sides, with your elbows completely bent, and make a fist with your hands.

5. Lift your left arm up beside your ear and bend as far to the right as possible, shifting your weight into a deep side lunge.

6. Rest your right arm on your thigh, giving slight support to your torso.

7. Keep lengthening your spine as you straighten up and return to the starting position. Never release this lengthening motion of your spine as you lower your spine into the side bend or as you lift your torso out of the side bend.

8. This should take 5 seconds to bend sideways and 5 seconds to return to the starting position.

9. Repeat on the other side.

10. Alternating sides, repeat 8 times.

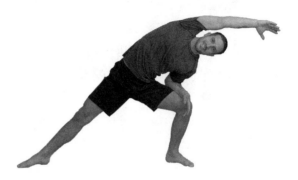

LEGS

# KICKS INTO SQUASH LUNGES

**Use visualization to stimulate your neurons:** Imagine playing squash and lunging as you move around the court. When doing a squash lunge, imagine that there are babies crawling around your feet. Be careful not to step on them! This will force you to land carefully and not just drop into a lunge in a sloppy manner.

**This sequence will** strengthen your hips, spine, and quads. It will align your connective tissue from the soles of your feet to your hips and increase your strength and energy as you move around in your daily life. It will also relieve and/or prevent hip and knee pain. It will increase your agility, giving you a bounce in your step.

**You should be feeling the work** in your hips, knees, and feet.

> If you suffer from chronic knee pain, bend your knees only as far as you are capable of before triggering the pain message. To heal knee pain, you must bend your knees, but it's important that you not go into the pain mode. You should find that your pain disappears quite rapidly when you are bending your knees just enough but not too much.

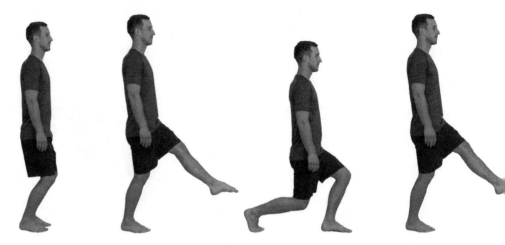

**Side View**

1. Place your feet together, bend your knees, straighten your spine, and allow your arms to hang by your sides.

2. Lift your left leg about a foot off the floor while straightening your right leg. Make sure not to lift your hip while lifting your left leg.

3. Hold your left leg in the air for 3 seconds to strengthen your balance.

4. Shift your weight into a squash lunge, moving your full body forward in space to keep the spine completely straight.

5. As you land in your squash lunge, imagine you are pulling your spine upward so that you land lightly on your foot.

6. Make sure that you land on the entire sole of the foot, not rolling in or out. This will ensure clean alignment, which will protect your joints from damage.

7. Bend your right knee, trying to keep it aligned with your torso and hip.

8. The squash lunge position is a quad stretch for the back leg, which is why it is important to keep your back straight and your bum pushing forward. As you do the exercise, play with the position to make sure you feel this quad stretch.

9. Lift the right heel off the floor, permitting the toes to be stretched as they remain on the floor.

10. Push yourself out of this position, returning your weight to your right leg and lifting the left leg in the air again.

11. Hold the lifted left leg for 3 seconds without rounding your back or lifting your hip. This is good for your balance.

12. Return to the starting position.

13. Repeat 4 times before changing legs.

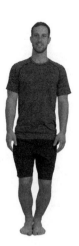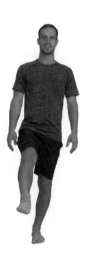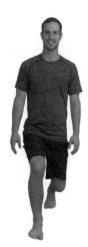

**Front View**

Remember, the chair is meant to prevent you from losing your balance. Do not grip it tightly or bend forward over it.

### FEET

**These four exercises for the feet will** increase the health and mobility of the ligaments, tendons, and muscles of your feet. In doing so, they will improve the alignment of your skeleton, starting from your feet and right up into your spine. By liberating your feet and improving mobility, you are starting the process of improving your posture and relieving conditions of arthritis in your feet, knees, and hips. Do not underestimate the value of these simple exercises. These are massively important, as the feet are the foundation of your entire body—and they govern your balance. When your feet are poorly aligned or weak, your body is prone to suffer from joint pain, arthritis, the need of joint replacements, and poor posture.

**Use visualization to stimulate your neurons:** Picture the skeleton of your foot and imagine each and every joint moving individually among the 28 bones in your foot.

**You should be feeling the work** in your toes, ankles, shins, and calves.

# TOE AND ANKLE PLIABILITY

1. Stand facing the back of your chair with your feet in a natural position (turned out or parallel, depending on your anatomy).
2. If you have good balance, hold the chair with one hand. Otherwise, hold it with both hands for more stability. In either case, don't let go of the chair, because your muscles will remain more relaxed when there is no need to worry about balance.
3. Lift your right heel as high as you can, leaving the ball of your foot and the first 3 toes flat on the floor.
4. Make sure the knee and the big toe are aligned.

5. Hold that position as you try to lift the heel a fraction higher for 3 to 4 seconds.

6. Push the toes against the floor in order to point the foot as much as possible, lifting the knee slightly higher.

7. Reverse the exercise by putting the toes back on the floor, keeping the heel raised.

8. Imagine you are squeezing an orange with your heel as you lower it. This will slow down the movement and build tension in your calf muscle.

9. Repeat 4 times before changing feet.

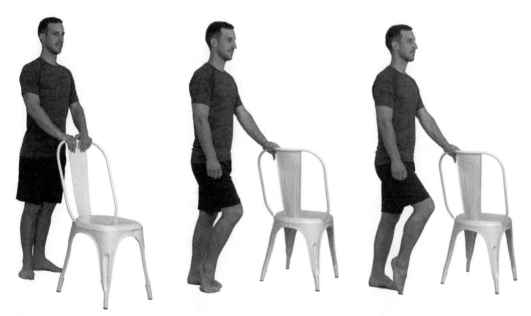

**Optional**

# TOE AND ANKLE PLIABILITY WITH LEG EXTENDED

1. Stand facing the back of your chair with your feet in a natural position (turned out or parallel, depending on your anatomy).

2. If you have good balance, hold the chair with one hand. Otherwise, hold it with both hands for more stability. If you need to hold it with both hands, turn slightly away from the chair to avoid hitting it with your foot. In either case, don't let go of the chair, because your muscles will remain more relaxed when there is no need to worry about balance.

3. Extend your right leg in front, keeping the knees straight.

4. Point your toes while keeping the foot close to the floor.

5. Keep your back straight; make sure that you do not lean back, sink in your hips, or round your lower back throughout the exercise.

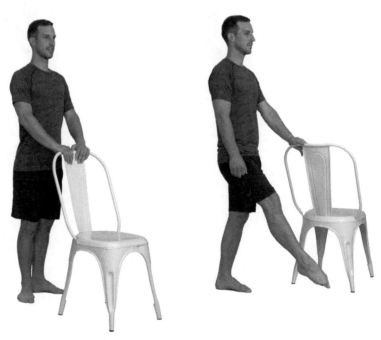

**Optional**

6. Flex your toes as much as possible, holding for 3 seconds as you continue to increase the toe flexion.

7. Flex your ankle as much as possible, holding for 3 seconds as you continue to increase the ankle flexion.

8. Reverse the exercise by flexing the toes for 3 seconds while pointing the ankle. This takes some coordination at first.

9. Point your toes for 3 seconds.

10. Finish by bringing your feet together in the starting position.

11. This sequence should take about 15 seconds.

12. Repeat 4 times before changing legs. This should take about 1 minute per leg.

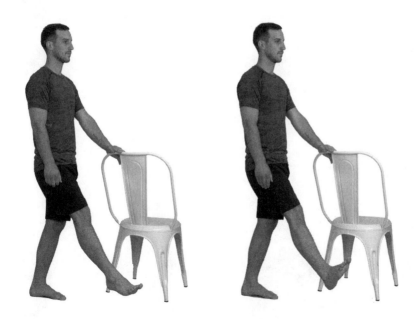

# SHIN STRETCHES FOR ANKLE MOBILITY, EXERCISE 1

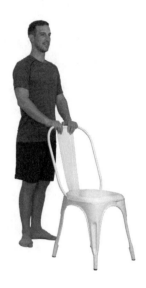

1. Stand facing the back of your chair with your feet together in a natural position (turned out or parallel, depending on your anatomy).

2. If you have good balance, hold the chair with one hand. Otherwise, hold it with both hands for more stability. In either case, don't let go of the chair, because your muscles will remain more relaxed when there is no need to worry about balance.

3. Bend your knees while keeping your back completely straight.

4. Raise your heels as high as possible, keeping the weight on the balls of your feet. Be careful to avoid ankle torsion, which occurs if you drop the weight on the baby toes.

5. Keeping the heels as high as possible, try to straighten your knees. As you do this, you will feel a deep stretch in your shins. This will increase your ankle flexibility.

6. Slowly lower your heels and bend your knees.

7. Repeat 4 times. Each repetition should take about 15 seconds.

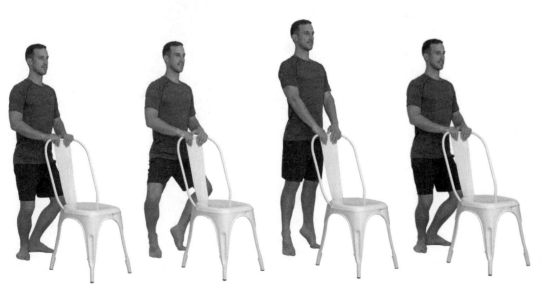

# SHIN STRETCHES FOR ANKLE MOBILITY, EXERCISE 2

1. Stand facing the back of your chair with your feet wider than hip-width distance apart (turned out or parallel, depending on your anatomy) and holding the chair with both hands.

2. Bend your knees while keeping your back completely straight.

3. Raise your heels as high as possible, keeping the weight on the balls of your feet. Be careful to avoid ankle torsion, which occurs if you drop the weight on the baby toes.

4. Keeping the heels as high as possible, try to straighten your knees. As you do this, you will feel a deep stretch in your shins. This will increase your ankle flexibility.

5. Slowly lower your heels and bend your knees.

6. Repeat 4 times. Each repetition should take about 15 seconds.

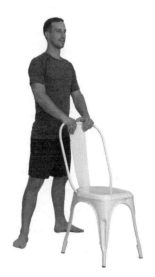

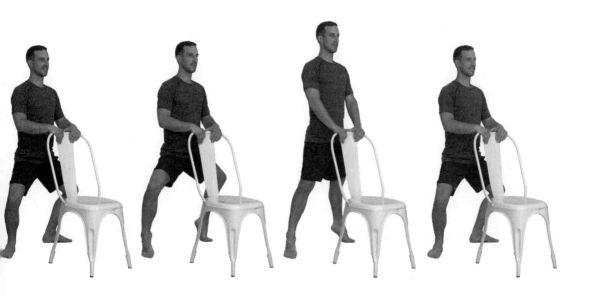

HIPS AND LEGS

# HIP STRETCHES

Please note that this stretch is the same as the one you did in Workout (on page 263).

**Use visualization to stimulate your neurons:** Imagine that you are rocking your hips in a hammock.

**This sequence will** relieve back pain, increase mobility in the connective tissue of your lower back and hips, and remove any connective tissue debris from the hip socket.

**You should be feeling the work** in your hips.

1. Stand next to your chair, holding it with your left hand.
2. Place your right foot flat on the seat of the chair, making sure that your full foot is flat on the seat. Bend your left leg.
3. Rest your right hand comfortably on your right thigh or knee, but don't force your knee to open with your hand.
4. Start rocking your hips from side to side. Move slowly so that you can go as far as possible to one side before rocking your hips to the other side.
5. Repeat the rocking motion 6 times, each time trying to swing your hips a little further.
6. Walk around the chair to the other side and repeat on the other leg.

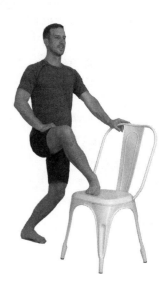

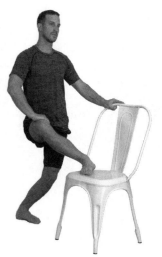

# PSOAS AND QUAD STRETCHES

**Use visualization to stimulate your neurons:** Imagine your hips as a wheel that you are continuously turning in order to round the lower spine.

**This sequence will** relieve back pain by rebalancing the muscles and connective tissue of the hip flexor group, composed of your psoas and quads. This muscle group is known for causing back pain and stiffness when imbalanced.

**You should be feeling the work** in the front of your hips and in your quads.

1. Stand facing the side of your chair, with your left hand holding the chair and your left foot flat on the seat.

2. Your right leg should be slightly behind you with the heel flat on the ground.

3. Lift the heel of your right leg and bend the knee.

4. Lock your tailbone in place, thinking of your hips as a wheel that you are rotating until you can't tuck your tailbone any further, and try to return the heel of your right leg to the floor. Count to 4 as you try to return your heel to the floor. If you lock your tailbone tight enough in its tucked-under position, it should be extremely difficult to put your heel flat on the floor. This is the psoas portion of the stretch.

5. Lift your right heel and bend your knee, pulling it close to the chair and tucking your tailbone under as much as possible.

6. Slowly lower your right knee to feel the quad stretch.

7. Go as far toward the floor as you can with no pain. The moment you reach your maximum, return immediately to the starting position. Do not hold the stretch; holding the stretch will have the effect of tightening your muscles.

8. Repeat 3 times before changing legs. This should take you 1 minute per side.

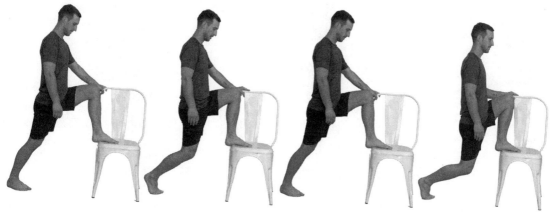

# HAMSTRING STRETCH WITH WINDMILL ARM

**Use visualization to stimulate your neurons:** Imagine your arm is the blade of a windmill as it draws a 360-degree circle.

**This sequence will** relieve back pain and improve posture by rebalancing the muscles and connective tissue of your spine, glutes, and hamstrings. It will also increase the range of motion of your hips, bringing energy and a feeling of effortlessness to movements like walking and running.

**You should be feeling the work** in your back, chest, and hamstrings.

1. Stand facing the side of your chair, holding the back of the chair with your left hand.
2. Place your left heel on the seat of the chair while reaching as high as you can with your right arm. Make sure you don't lift your right hip while you do this.
3. Start the windmill by pulling your right arm over the leg on the chair. You will feel this stretch in both your hamstrings and your back muscles. If it is too difficult to keep the knee on the chair straight, feel free to bend it.

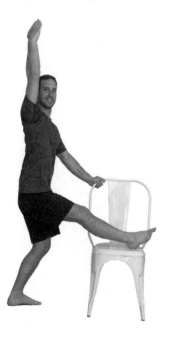
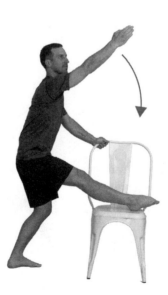
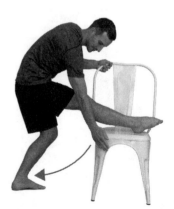

4. Continue the windmill motion, sweeping the arm toward the floor as you let your back round.

5. As you pull your arm toward the floor, sweep past your right ankle and twist your torso toward the back of the room.

6. Raise your arm above your head to where you started the windmill.

7. One complete windmill should take 20 seconds.

8. Repeat 3 times per leg before changing legs. This is an extremely deep stretch, so shake out before switching legs.

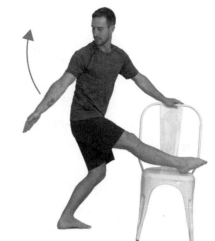

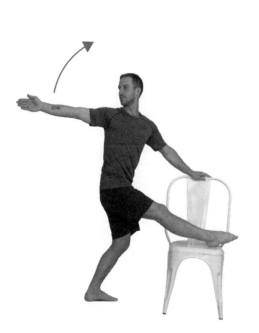

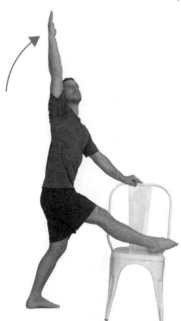

SPINE

# STANDING SPINE STRETCH WITH WINDMILL ARM

**Use visualization to stimulate your neurons:** Imagine your arm is the blade of a windmill as it draws a 360-degree circle.

**This sequence will** relieve back pain and improve posture by rebalancing the muscles and connective tissue of your spine. It will also increase the range of motion of your spine, bringing energy and a feeling of effortlessness to your daily activities, such as dressing yourself, or fun activities, such as playing tennis and golf.

**You should be feeling the work** in your back and chest.

1. Stand next to the back of your chair, holding it with your left hand and relaxing your right arm at your side.

2. Place your right foot directly in front of your left foot, making sure that the soles of your feet are flat on the ground and not rolling in or out at your ankles. You may have to adjust the placement of your feet in order to keep them flat on the ground.

**Front View**

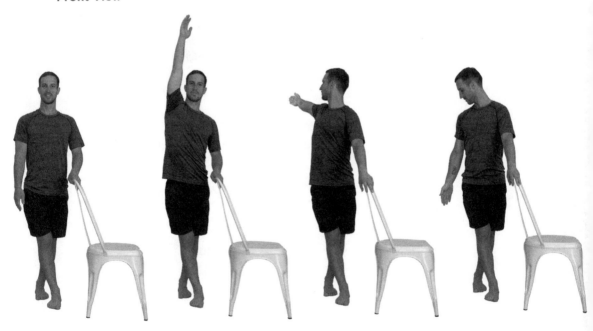

3. Raise your right arm in front of you as you begin to slowly draw a full 360-degree circle.

4. Continue raising your arm overhead and behind you, twisting your spine as much as possible to stretch all of the muscles of your spine.

5. Continue lowering your arm until you arrive at your starting position, with your arm resting at your side.

6. Each windmill should take 15 seconds to complete.

7. Repeat 4 times before changing arms.

**Side View**

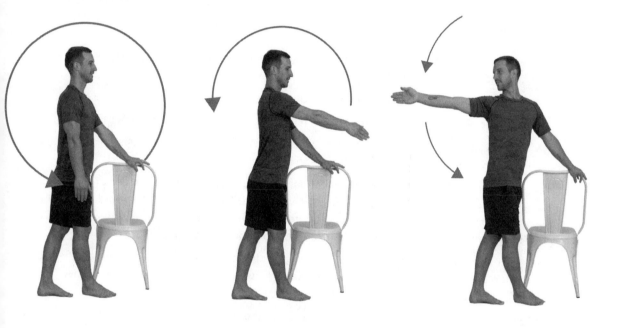

# FULL SPINE STRETCHES

**Use visualization to stimulate your neurons:** Imagine your back alternates between being flat like a tabletop and curved up like a cat's spine when it stretches. During this exercise, you will play between a rounded spine and a tabletop flat spine.

**This sequence will** relieve tension throughout the muscles and connective tissue of your back, from your shoulders through your hips. It will elongate your spine, open up the pectoral muscles to improve your posture, and reverse spine shrinkage.

**You should be feeling the work** in your shoulder blades, spine, hips, hamstrings, inner thigh muscles (adductors), and glutes.

1. Stand facing the back of your chair, holding the chair with both hands shoulder-width distance apart.
2. Walk back from the chair until your elbows fully extend. Your back should be flat.
3. Your feet should be placed wider than hip-width distance apart, with your knees bent.
4. Once you've arrived in this position, relax your shoulder blades to assist in stretching your arms farther to help release tension in the chest muscles.
5. Shift your weight gently from side to side, to release tension on both sides of the spine. This relaxed mini side-to-side shifting should take 10 seconds. This should feel really good. It shouldn't hurt. Move the way a cat does when it stretches its spine. Allow your spine to articulate throughout the exercise; don't hold it straight.
6. Shift into deeper spine stretches by straightening one knee and bending the other as you round your back. The entire time, keep moving your spine from side to side. This will really loosen up the spine muscles.
7. Take 6 seconds before shifting your weight to the other leg.
8. Repeat 2 times per side.
9. Return your weight to both legs, to the center, with a rounded back.
10. Slowly try to straighten your knees. This will stretch your hamstrings and back muscles.
11. Slowly bend and straighten your knees 4 times. It doesn't matter if you can't fully straighten your knees or your back. Never force a stretch.

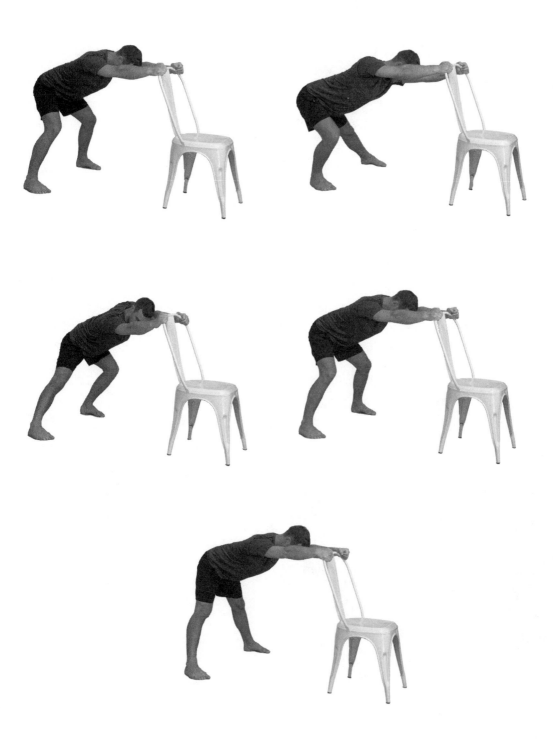

# FLEXION AND EXTENSION OF THE UPPER BACK AND NECK

**Use visualization to stimulate your neurons:** Imagine a string attached to the center of your skull that is pulling you upward as you lift your face toward the ceiling. When you move your head, always visualize it moving up and out of your shoulders. Your neck will be in a constant state of elongation.

**This sequence will** relieve tension throughout the muscles and connective tissue of your upper back, including your neck, chest, and shoulders. It will elongate your spine, open up the pectoral muscles to improve your posture, and reverse spine shrinkage. It is excellent for reducing headaches.

**You should be feeling the work** in both the front and the back of your neck and pectorals.

1. Stand facing the back of your chair, holding the chair with both hands.
2. Position your feet in parallel and comfortably placed on the floor, slightly wider than hip-width distance apart. Do not force your feet to turn in or out.

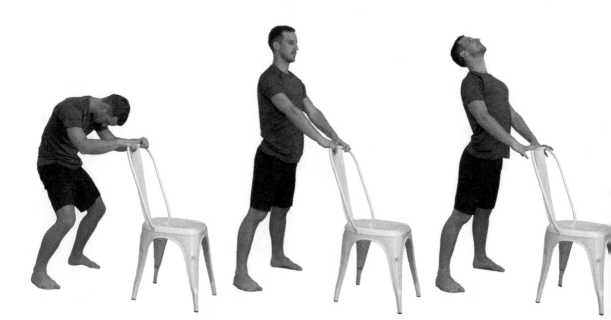

3. Bend both knees, round your back in a Neutral C (see page 111), and let your head lean forward so that it stays in line with your neck.

4. Round your spine, making sure that your lower back is as tucked under as possible and that your shoulders do not drop beyond your knees. Do not stick your bum out or arch your back, as this will compress your spine rather than stretch it.

5. Straighten your legs, spine, and neck, looking straight in front of you.

6. Open your chest as wide as you can while imagining you are dropping your shoulders in your back pocket as your upper back slightly arches.

7. As you arch your back, let your chest open while lifting your face toward the ceiling. Do not release your neck muscles, keeping your head well supported as you pull your skull upward.

8. Be aware of not sinking into your lower spine while slightly arching your upper back. Sinking into your lower back often involves pushing your hips forward and letting your spine drop downward.

9. The moment you cannot go any farther, straighten your neck, looking in front of you, and then return to the starting position with your knees bent and head forward.

10. This entire sequence should take 20 seconds.

11. Repeat 4 times.

# NECK PLIABILITY

**Use visualization to stimulate your neurons:** Imagine a string attached to the center of your skull that is pulling your neck upward as you move your head in various directions. When you move your head, always visualize it moving up and out of your shoulders. Your neck will be in a constant state of elongation.

**This sequence will** relieve tension throughout the muscles and connective tissue of your neck. It will elongate your neck and improve your posture, while relieving headaches and back pain.

**You should be feeling the work** in the front, back, and sides of your neck.

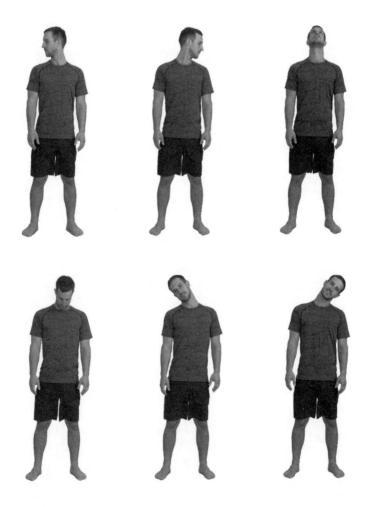

### Sequence 1

1. Stand with your feet hip-width distance apart, arms relaxed at your sides and back straight.

2. Rotate your head to the right, trying to put your chin over your right shoulder. Don't let your shoulder go up.

3. Hold this position for 6 seconds before switching to the other side.

4. Alternating sides, repeat 8 times.

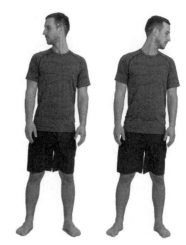

### Sequence 2

1. Stand with your feet hip-width distance apart, arms relaxed at your sides and back straight.

2. Raise and lower your head, pulling up on the neck vertebrae as you do each movement so as never to compress your neck joints or discs.

3. Take 6 seconds to raise your head and 6 seconds to lower it. This counts as 1 repetition.

4. Repeat 4 times.

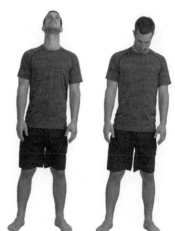

### Sequence 3

1. Stand with your feet hip-width distance apart, arms relaxed at your sides and back straight.

2. Tilt your head sideways as far as you can without moving your torso or shoulders.

3. Take 6 seconds to tilt your head in one direction before switching to the other side.

4. Repeat 8 times, counting a tilt to both sides as 1 repetition.

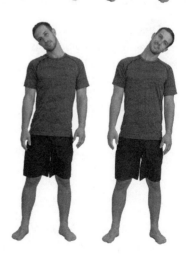

## PART TWO OF WORKOUT 3: Floor Exercises (Optional)

### ABDOMINALS

The next three exercises are sit-ups to engage your abdominal muscles. Remember:

- When doing sit-ups, do not press the center of your spine into the floor, as is traditionally taught. Pressing it into the floor actually damages the spine and can lead to slipped and bulging discs.
- Use this trick to help you identify the muscles to engage in a sit-up: lie on your back with your knees bent. Put your hands between your pubic bone and your hipbones and cough. When you cough, you will feel your transverse abdominis muscles contract. Those are the ones we want to engage, as they are crucial in strengthening and flattening your stomach.
- When you lift your shoulders off the floor, imagine that you are pulling your pubic bone and your ribs toward each other. Never do a sit-up by leading with your head and using the head and neck to pull the upper body off the floor. This will cause neck damage and headaches and will do little to strengthen your stomach.
- As you do your sit-up, move very slowly so that you use nothing but your muscles to lift you off the floor. Do not use momentum or speed to lift off the floor rapidly. Slow movement is more effective in strengthening your muscles.
- Your head will naturally be lifted off the floor as your shoulders rise up. Because you are not pulling with your head, your chin will not drop toward your chest and your face will remain looking at the ceiling.
- By keeping your head aligned with your spine during the sit-ups, you will protect your neck from injury.

This sequence will strengthen your abdominal and oblique muscles, as well as the muscles of your spine. This will increase the strength and flexibility of your upper spine into the ribs and the full shoulder girdle. It will help you to maintain good posture.

You should be feeling the work in your rectus abdominis, transverse abdominis, obliques, and psoas.

> If you have a rounded back that prevents you from maintaining clean alignment when lying on the floor, place a firm cushion under your head. This will straighten the spine and avoid compression in your neck.

# RAISED ARM SIT-UPS

1. Lie flat on the ground, knees bent, feet placed flat on the ground, hip-width distance apart.

2. Place your right hand behind your head, fingers barely touching your head, while opening your right elbow as wide as possible.

3. Raise your left arm to the ceiling.

4. Following the notes on page 332 on abdominal exercises, contract your abs to raise your upper back. Reach toward the ceiling with your left hand, permitting your body to twist in order to raise the arm higher. Count 3 seconds to raise and 3 seconds to lower.

5. Exhale when you contract your abs to lift and twist, and inhale as you lower.

6. Maintain control of your stomach muscles the entire time, making sure not to relax them or hold them in extreme tension.

7. Repeat 16 times before switching sides.

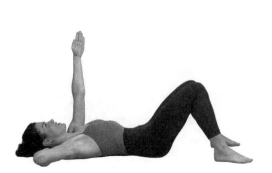 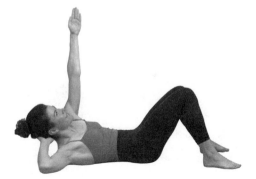

# TOUCH THE KNEE SIT-UPS

1. Lie flat on the ground, knees bent, feet placed flat on the ground hip-width distance apart.

2. Place your right hand behind your head, fingers barely touching, while opening your right elbow as wide as possible.

3. Raise the left arm toward the opposite knee.

4. Following the notes on page 332 on abdominal exercises, contract your abs to raise your upper back. Try to touch the fingers of your left hand to the right knee, permitting your body to twist in order to raise yourself up higher. Count 3 seconds to raise and 3 seconds to lower.

5. Exhale when you contract your abs to lift and twist, and inhale as you lower.

6. Maintain control of your stomach muscles the entire time, making sure not to relax them or hold them in extreme tension.

7. Repeat 16 times before switching sides.

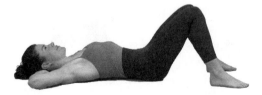 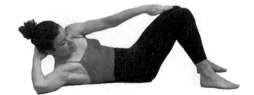

# SIDE BEND SIT-UPS

1. Lie flat on the ground, knees bent, feet placed flat on the ground hip-width distance apart.

2. Place your left hand behind your head, fingers barely touching, while opening your left elbow as wide as possible.

3. Raise the right arm 1 inch off of the floor.

4. Following the notes on page 334 on abdominal exercises, contract your abs to raise your upper back.

5. Slide your right arm toward your right ankle, permitting your body to bend sideways. Count 3 seconds to bend and 3 seconds to return to a straight spine.

6. Exhale when you contract your abs to lift and bend, and inhale as you return.

7. Maintain control of your stomach muscles the entire time, making sure not to relax them or grip them in extreme tension.

8. Repeat 16 times before switching sides.

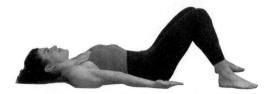 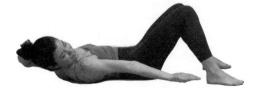

LEGS

The next four exercises comprise a side-leg series. Do all four exercises on one leg before switching to the other leg.

**Use visualization to stimulate your neurons:** Imagine pulling your leg out of the hip socket during the entire exercise. Also, imagine that you are being pulled from the top of your head in one direction and the tips of your toes in the other.

**This sequence will** strengthen your hips and full core while slenderizing and toning your legs and glutes. It will hydrate and reinforce the crimp in the ligaments of the hips, knees, and spine, giving you strength and balance.

**You should be feeling the work** in your hips, glutes, spine, inner thighs, ribs, waist, and back (if you are correctly lengthening your muscles throughout the exercise).

# DOUBLE-LEG AND TRUNK LIFT

1. Lie on your right side, with both legs extended, toes pointed, and knees straight.

2. Straighten your right arm and extend it on the ground, resting your head gently on it. Do not put your head in your hand because it is bad for your neck.

3. Important: Place your left arm in front of your shoulder for additional support.

4. Squeeze your feet together and lift both legs off the floor while lifting your trunk in a side crunch.

5. Take 3 seconds to lift the legs and torso and 3 seconds to lower them.

6. Repeat 8 times with pointed feet.

7. Stay on this side to do the following exercises.

> Make side leg lifts more comfortable by placing your hip in the hole of a firm hemorrhoid cushion (not the inflatable kind).

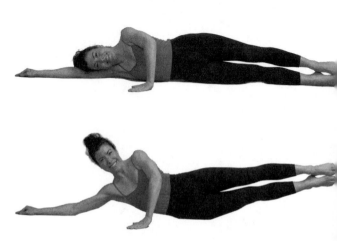

# SCISSORS

1. Continuing from the starting position in the previous exercise, lift your left leg while keeping the right leg flat on the ground.

2. Bring both legs together in a scissor action, with the upper leg lowering midway and the lower leg raising up to join it.

3. Take 3 seconds to scissor the legs together and 1 second to open them.

4. Repeat 8 times.

5. Stay on this side to do the following exercises.

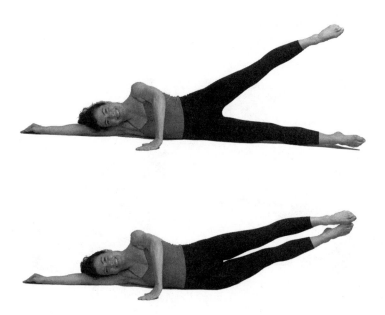

# SIDE LEG LIFTS AND CIRCLES

1. Continuing on the same side from the previous exercise, bend your right knee and extend the left leg sideways with pointed toes.

2. Bend your right arm, placing the forearm directly under your shoulder so that it acts as a support for your torso.

3. Important: Place your left arm in front for additional support.

4. Slide your left foot along the floor away from the body, lifting it when you can't slide any farther. This makes the leg feel very heavy; however, this will strengthen and slenderize your legs.

5. Take 3 seconds to lift the leg and 3 seconds to lower it.

6. Repeat 8 times with a pointed foot, and 8 times with a flexed foot.

7. Draw a circle with your left foot, 4 times forward and 4 times backward, with a pointed foot.

8. Repeat drawing circles with a flexed foot.

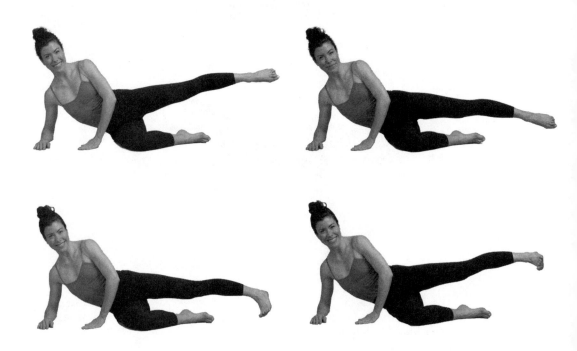

# QUAD STRETCH

1. Continuing on the same side from the previous exercise, keep your right knee bent.

2. Bend your left leg behind you and take the ankle of the left leg with your hand or a stretch band and try to pull the ankle close to your bum.

3. Take 3 seconds to pull the knee toward your bum and 3 seconds to release it.

4. Repeat 4 times on this leg.

Take 30 seconds to shake out the tension from your hips and legs before changing sides. Once you've changed sides, start the 4-exercise side-leg series sequence from the beginning.

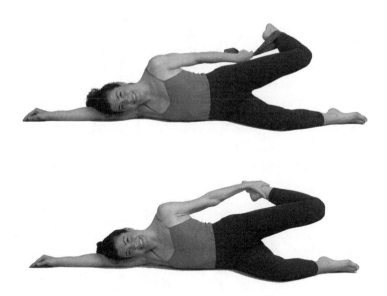

DEEP STRETCHES

# HAMSTRING STRETCH

**This sequence will** stretch the connective tissue and muscles of your glutes and hamstrings. It will increase your energy, give you a wider stride as you walk and run, help reduce tightness in your back, and improve your posture.

**You should be feeling the work** in your hamstrings and glutes.

---

- If you have a rounded back that prevents you from maintaining clean alignment when lying on the floor, place a firm cushion under your head. This will straighten the spine and avoid compression in your neck.

- If you have trouble holding on to your leg without lifting your back off the floor, use a stretch band or a towel to avoid raising your back off the floor and straining your neck. Raising your back also interferes with your ability to release the muscles into a stretch.

---

1. Lie flat on the ground with your left knee bent and the sole of the foot flat on the ground.
2. Raise your right leg.
3. Hold the right leg with both hands beneath the thigh. Use a stretch band or towel if needed.
4. Take 6 seconds to bend the right knee, pulling it toward your chest.

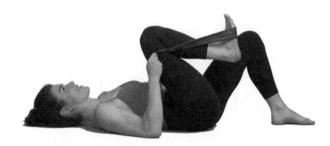

5. Take 6 seconds as you try to straighten the right knee. Most people cannot straighten their knee. You will feel this stretch in your hamstrings.

6. Take 6 seconds to bend the knee again and pull the leg toward your chest, while wiggling your bum slowly 4 times.

7. Take 6 seconds as you try again to straighten the right knee.

8. Repeat bending the knee, wiggling the bum, and straightening the knee once more before changing legs.

9. Repeat the entire sequence on the other leg.

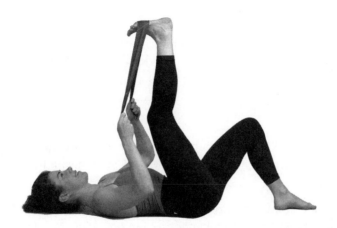

# SEATED IT BAND STRETCH

Please note that this stretch is similar to the one you did in Workout 2.

This sequence will stretch the IT band, a wide strip of connective tissue that runs down the length of the outer thigh, from the top of the pelvis to the shin. When it becomes tight, it causes arthritis in the knee, chronic knee pain, and possibly the need for knee replacement.

You should be feeling the work in the outside of your thighs. You may feel a minor discomfort near your knee. As long as it is not a sharp pain, do not worry.

> If you have tight hamstring or back muscles, sit on a riser. Use a stretch band if you have trouble reaching your foot.

1. Sit on the floor with both legs extended. If your hamstrings are tight, you may not be able to straighten your knees. Do not worry; this will still stretch your hamstrings.

2. Point your left foot and flex your right foot.

3. Place your left hand across your right leg or wrap a stretch band around your ankle, holding it with your left hand while simultaneously twisting your spine to the right.

4. Place your right hand on the floor behind you, using it to help keep your spine straight. Do not round your spine during this exercise.

5. With the fingers of your left hand, walk down the outside your right leg as far as you can, keeping your back straight and your right foot as flexed as possible.

6. Hold for 6 seconds.

7. Return to your starting position and relax your leg.

8. Repeat 4 times before switching legs.

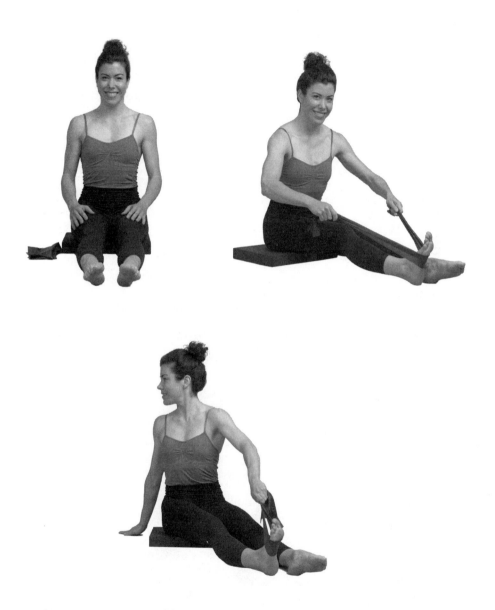

# SEATED SPINE STRETCHES

**Use visualization to stimulate your neurons:** Imagine the muscles of your shoulder blades, shoulders, and full spine are being gently kneaded in a self-massage.

**This sequence will** release tension in your spine through stretching and strengthening. The combination of this exercise and the previous one will rebalance all of the connective tissue and muscles of your spine. It will improve your posture and relieve back pain.

**You should be feeling the work** in your ribs, shoulder blades, triceps, lower back, hips, and glutes.

> If you have tight hamstrings or back muscles, sit on a riser.

1. Sit on the floor with both legs bent and the soles of your feet flat on the floor.
2. Your feet should be placed wider than hip-width distance apart.
3. Your spine should be straight and pulling upward to the maximum of your ability. Look straight in front of you.
4. Raise your shoulders as high as you can, pulling upward with your spine and holding on tightly to your knees.

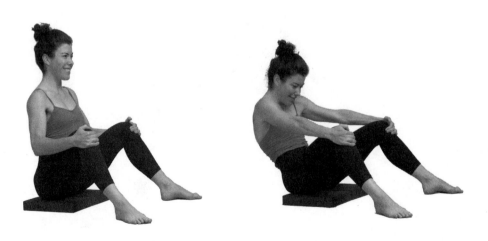

5. Take 3 seconds to slowly let your weight drop backward as you imagine that you are rolling down vertebra by vertebra as you go. Don't crunch the vertebrae but lift out of your spine as you drop backward.

6. Take one knee with both hands and move around gently, swaying from the base of your spine up through the shoulder blades and into the shoulders. This should take you 10 seconds. Make sure your shoulders are raised as high as possible. Repeat on the other knee.

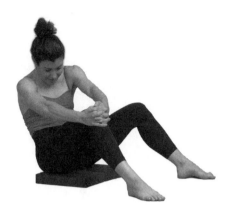

7. Return to your starting position, rolling up one vertebra at a time until you are sitting completely straight, shoulders down, elbows pulled in toward your ribs. This should take 3 seconds.

8. Lift your chin toward the ceiling, pulling the individual discs of your neck apart. This should take 6 seconds.

9. Return to the starting position, looking straight in front.

10. Repeat 3 times.

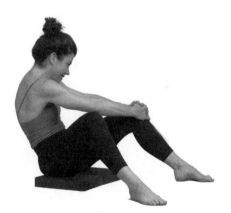
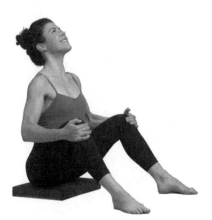

# CHAPTER 12

# FOR EVERYONE

### *Daily Mini-Workouts to Amplify Your Fast Track*

These eight brief but spectacular mini-workouts will take you a maximum of 1 to 2 minutes to do. I suggest you sprinkle these exercises throughout each day during your 30-day challenge and beyond. Do them as often as you'd like, and eventually you will find yourself automatically doing them while you're on the bus, doing laundry, or having a conversation. Constant movement is the objective. These are easy to do discreetly so that no one will think that you are distracted, and they're fun to do in unconventional places, like at the theater. They are very simple, but by doing them throughout every day you will give your Fast Track program a little power boost—and create a habit of moving throughout your day.

I swear by them. I do them in meetings, sitting at my computer, standing around talking, in the kitchen, as I am waiting in line at a store. I do finger, wrist, and shoulders stretches discreetly. I do them because it feels good. I firmly believe that constant movement is a large part of why I am in such good shape! Life should be a mini-workout.

A good way to remind yourself to do these mini-workouts is to put Post-its on your fridge, bathroom mirror, or the remote control. After a few weeks, you will find yourself wiggling your fingers and toes without having to be reminded to do it.

## MINI-WORKOUT 1: FOR FINGER AND WRIST MOBILITY

Do these movements as often as you'd like:

- Rotate your wrists in both directions.
- Flex and extend your wrists up and down.
- Make a tight fist and open your fingers as wide as possible.
- Pretend to play the piano by moving one finger at a time.

These exercises will not hurt you and will help relieve the pain of arthritis, as well as shoulder and neck pain. (They also help relieve migraines!)

## MINI-WORKOUT 2: FOR TOE AND ANKLE MOBILITY

Do as many of the toe and ankle isolation exercises as you can:

- Point your feet, flex your toes, then flex your ankles, then reverse it.
- Extend your ankles while keeping your toes flexed, then point your toes.
- Rotate your ankles slowly, and in both directions.

## MINI-WORKOUT 3: FOR SPINE FLEXIBILITY

During your first trip to the bathroom in the morning, place one hand on the side of the vanity or sink, position your feet wide apart, and twist your spine in the opposite direction of your hand, trying to turn your full torso so you can look behind you. (You can do this in the kitchen, holding on to the kitchen counter, or at work, holding on to your desk.)

## MINI-WORKOUT 4: FOR SPINE LENGTHENING

This is another one to do during that first bathroom trip. Standing at the sink, reach above your head with one arm and try to "touch" the ceiling (not literally, but reach far!) with your fingers. Slowly alternate your arms with each ceiling reach, repeating 16 times. Doing this in the morning will get your posture set for the day and help stop spine shrinkage.

## MINI-WORKOUT 5: FOR ELBOW RELAXATION

This can be done at any time—standing on the bus, chatting with a friend, or sitting at your desk. Bend your elbows and quickly straighten them, imagining you are flicking water off your fingers, as if you just washed your hands. This will force your elbows to relax, which indirectly helps the shoulders and neck to relax.

## MINI-WORKOUT 6: FOR CIRCULATION

Before you sit down to watch TV or start work, take a moment to do this mini-workout. From a standing position, take side-to-side steps, alternating sides 16 times, to get the blood circulating and increasing your energy level before beginning your next task.

## MINI-WORKOUT 7: FOR RELEASING NECK AND HEAD TENSION

Try to do this movement all of the time, during a conversation or while working, spending time on the computer, or watching TV. Slowly and in a relaxed mode, remember to keep turning your head and raising and lowering your chin. Try not to ever just sit looking straight in front of you for an extended period of time.

## MINI-WORKOUT 8: FOR STRENGTHENING AND STRETCHING YOUR CALVES

Do these heel raisers while waiting for the kettle to boil. Steady yourself by holding on to the kitchen counter, wall, or handrail while you slowly raise and lower your heels. Don't worry about the height you raise your heels—even a little bit is good for you. Do a maximum of 8 heel raisers at a time, and wait at least an hour before doing another set of 8.

# CHAPTER 13

# MARK THE CHANGE: CELEBRATE YOUR PROGRESS ON DAY 1, DAY 15, AND DAY 30

There is nothing like the thrill of seeing the proof of your improved strength and flexibility in black and white. Take these fitness evaluations on Day 1, Day 15, and Day 30 of the Fast Track plan and record how you are getting younger.

> Don't forget to take the Mirror Test (page 116) on Day 1 and Day 30, too.

## THE STAIR TEST

The goal of this test is to check how easily you can climb stairs, not to win a race.

Set a timer for 5 minutes to see how many stairs you can climb up and down in that time.

# TRACK YOUR PROGRESS

1. *How many steps were you able to take in five minutes?*
   DAY 1: _____        DAY 15: _____        DAY 30: _____

2. *Did you feel unsteady, as if you would fall, while you were stepping up and down?*
   (Circle a number from 0 to 5, with 0 meaning you felt steady and balanced, 5 meaning you felt unsteady and as though you might fall.)
   0     1     2     3     4     5

3. *Average pain level*
   (Circle a number from 0 to 5, with 0 meaning no pain and 5 meaning the worst imaginable pain.)
   0     1     2     3     4     5

4. *If you were in pain, where did you feel it?*
   DAY 1:      _____
   DAY 15:     _____
   DAY 30:     _____

## THE GET UP AND GO TEST

The Get Up and Go Test measures the ease and effort it takes to get up, walk a short distance, and return to a seated position. This test is commonly used by physical and occupational therapists to assess a person's gait, walking ability, and balance. Performance on this test is also seen as a strong indicator of a person's mobility. Repeat the same sequence each time you take this test.

1. Choose a set distance, such as 10 feet (3 meters) away from a chair.
2. Set a timer (or ask someone to time you).
3. Sit with your back against the chair.
4. Rise from a sitting position.
5. Walk the set distance.
6. Turn around.
7. Return to the chair and sit down.
8. Turn off the timer.

# TRACK YOUR PROGRESS

1. *How long did it take you to complete the Get Up and Go Test?* (seconds)
   DAY 1: _____        DAY 15: _____        DAY 30: _____

2. *Did you use the support of an armrest, cane, table, or other to rise?* (Y/N)
   DAY 1: _____        DAY 15: _____        DAY 30: _____

3. *Did you feel unsteady, as if you would fall while you were getting up and down?*
   (Circle a number from 0 to 5, with 0 meaning you felt steady and balanced, 5 meaning you felt unsteady and as though you might fall.)
   0     1     2     3     4     5

4. *Average pain level* during *this exercise*
   (Circle a number from 0 to 5, with 0 meaning no pain and 5 the worst imaginable pain.)
   0     1     2     3     4     5

5. *Average pain level* after *this exercise*
   (Circle a number from 0 to 5, with 0 meaning no pain and 5 the worst imaginable pain.)
   0     1     2     3     4     5

6. *Where did you feel the pain?*
   DAY 1:       _____
   DAY 15:      _____
   DAY 30:      _____

## THE WALKING TEST

This is not a very accurate test, as some days we are more energetic than others, but it is fun to take anyway.

Walk the same route each time, noting where you were after 10 minutes. As you do this test, keep these guidelines in mind:

1. Set a timer for 10 minutes.
2. Begin walking.
3. Walk as far as possible in 10 minutes.

4. Stop the timer after 10 minutes and see how far you have gone compared to your previous walk.

# TRACK YOUR PROGRESS

1. *How much distance did you cover doing the Walking Test?* (miles/kilometers)

   DAY 1: _____        DAY 15: _____        DAY 30: _____

2. *Did you use the support of a cane or walking aid to complete this test?* (Y/N)

   DAY 1: _____        DAY 15: _____        DAY 30: _____

3. *Did you feel unsteady, as if you would fall while you were walking?*
   (Circle a number between 0 and 5, with 0 meaning you felt steady and balanced and 5 meaning you felt unsteady and as though you might fall.)

   0      1      2      3      4      5

4. *Average pain level* during *this exercise*
   (Circle a number from 0 to 5, with 0 meaning no pain and 5 the worst imaginable pain.)

   0      1      2      3      4      5

5. *Average pain level* after *this exercise*
   (Circle a number from 0 to 5, with 0 meaning no pain and 5 the worst imaginable pain.)

   0      1      2      3      4      5

6. *If you were in pain, where did you feel it?*

   DAY 1:        _____
   DAY 15:       _____
   DAY 30:       _____

## MOBILITY AND FLEXIBILITY TESTS

These four tests—the Stand and Reach Test, the Sock Test, the Back Touch Test, and the Lie Down, Sit Up, Get Up Test—help us to become more conscious of the status of our current mobility and flexibility and how they change during the 30-day program. The movements tested mirror the kinds of movements we do in our everyday life and are a good indicator of the current health and chronological age of our body.

They can be a good wake-up call to notice how we've adapted to our sedentary way of life.

### Stand and Reach Test

This test evaluates the range of motion in your shoulders and your overall functional mobility level for daily tasks; it tests the strength and flexibility of the muscles of your spine and torso. We have many muscles running along the spine that offer support within each vertebra. If these muscles start to degrade, we can develop conditions such as arthritis, osteoporosis, and frozen shoulder. The strength and flexibility of these muscle groups (such as the lattisimus dorsi, the deltoids, and the rotator cuff) can reduce pain in the back, neck, and shoulder areas. Freedom of movement and range of motion will help you in your daily life, such as reaching up into the cupboard or twisting to grab something off the back seat in the car.

Repeat the same variation each time you take this test. As you do this test, keep these guidelines in mind:

1. Stand facing a wall, about 1 foot away.
2. Extend your right arm up to touch the wall as high as you can.
3. Try reaching for something on the ceiling.
4. Use a pencil to mark how high you were able to reach.
5. Repeat with your other arm.

## TRACK YOUR PROGRESS

1. *How high could you reach while doing the Stand and Reach Test?*
   DAY 1: _____      DAY 15: _____      DAY 30: _____

2. *Average pain level* during *this exercise*
   (Circle a number from 0 to 5, with 0 meaning no pain and 5 the worst imaginable pain.)
   0      1      2      3      4      5

3. *Average pain level* after *this exercise*
   (Circle a number from 0 to 5, with 0 meaning no pain and 5 the worst imaginable pain.)
   0      1      2      3      4      5

4. *Where did you feel the pain?*

> DAY 1: _____
>
> DAY 15: _____
>
> DAY 30: _____

5. *How fatiguing was it to extend your arm upward?*
   (Circle a number from 0 to 5, with 0 meaning no fatigue and 5 meaning exhausted.)

   0     1     2     3     4     5

### The Sock Test

Putting our socks on can provide insight into the ways our body has changed with time. As deceptively simple as this act is, our ability to complete it can help us evaluate hip mobility, as well as many other things: overall strength, flexibility, range of motion, and motor control of your entire body. While there is no wrong and right way to put a sock on and take it off, doing this test can help you begin to analyze the ways in which your body may overcompensate or unconsciously avoid certain movements while completing a task. Use this test to become more conscious of this daily action; attach your mind to the movement.

1. Use a timer and start the timer when you begin.

2. Start with no socks on.

3. Put one sock on.

4. Put the other sock on.

5. Take the first sock off.

6. Take the other sock off.

7. Stop the timer.

## TRACK YOUR PROGRESS

1. *Was this easy to do? (Y/N)*

   > DAY 1: ____     DAY 15: ____     DAY 30: ____

2. *How fast were you able to get through this exercise?*

   > DAY 1: ____     DAY 15: ____     DAY 30: ____

3. *Average pain level* during *this exercise*
   (Circle a number from 0 to 5, with 0 meaning no pain and 5 the worst imaginable pain.)

   0    1    2    3    4    5

4. *Average pain level* after *this exercise*
   (Circle a number from 0 to 5, with 0 meaning no pain and 5 the worst imaginable pain.)

   0    1    2    3    4    5

## The Back Touch Test

By doing daily exercises that involve rebalancing the shoulder joints and the rotator cuff muscles, we protect our range of motion and help to decrease our risk of pain. As we age, we want to avoid problems before they arise; we want to avoid pain and retain mobility. The Back Touch Test will help you evaluate the strength and flexibility of your rib cage and shoulders—which govern your ability to dress and groom yourself, reach into the back seat, even go to the bathroom. This test will chart your improvement after doing your daily workouts.

1. Touch your left shoulder with your right hand.
2. Touch your right shoulder with your right hand.
3. Touch your right waist with your right hand.
4. Touch your right lower spine with your right hand.
5. Touch your left shoulder blade with your right hand.
6. Repeat the test on the other side with the other hand.

# TRACK YOUR PROGRESS

1. *Did you use the assistance of your other arm to be able to reach any part of your back?* (Y/N)

   DAY 1: _____        DAY 15: _____        DAY 30: _____

2. *Could you complete all the touches easily?* (Y/N)

   DAY 1: _____        DAY 15: _____        DAY 30: _____

3. *Average pain level* during *this exercise*
   (Circle a number from 0 to 5, with 0 meaning no pain and 5 the worst imaginable pain.)

   0     1     2     3     4     5

4. *Average pain level* after *this exercise*
   (Circle a number from 0 to 5, with 0 meaning no pain and 5 the worst imaginable pain.)

   0     1     2     3     4     5

5. *Were you limited in your range of motion?*

   DAY 1:     _____

   DAY 15:    _____

   DAY 30:    _____

## The Lie Down, Sit Up, Get Up Test

It's easy to take movement for granted. But when we can't get out of a chair easily or pick ourselves up off the floor, we're in dire shape. These actions require you to have strength, flexibility, and muscle power relative to the weight of your body—especially in your larger muscle groups, such as your quads, glutes, and core. These movements also require that you have balance and motor coordination.

This test will provide a lot of insight into your ability to perform simple daily activities, such as retrieving something that falls under the bed or getting into and out of the bathtub without falling. Studies have shown that the ability to lie down on and get back up off the floor is a predictor of your longevity and can also be a very accurate indicator of your ability to live an independent life.[20]

1. Start a timer.

2. From a standing position, lie down on the floor.

3. Get back up.

4. Turn off the timer.

# TRACK YOUR PROGRESS

1. *How long did it take you to lie down on the floor and get back up?*
   DAY 1: _____          DAY 15: _____          DAY 30: _____

2. *Did you use the assistance of a wall, chair, hands, or arms to be able to get down or up from the floor or the chair? (Y/N)*
   DAY 1: _____          DAY 15: _____          DAY 30: _____

3. *If yes, which ones and how did you use them?*
   DAY 1:          _____
   DAY 15:         _____
   DAY 30:         _____

4. *Was your movement coordinated and controlled? (Y/N)*
   DAY 1: _____          DAY 15: _____          DAY 30: _____

5. *Did you feel strong and confident during this exercise? (Y/N)*
   DAY 1: _____          DAY 15: _____          DAY 30: _____

6. *Average pain level during this exercise*
   (Circle a number from 0 to 5, with 0 meaning no pain and 5 the worst imaginable pain.)
   0     1     2     3     4     5

7. *Average pain level after this exercise*
   (Circle a number from 0 to 5, with 0 meaning no pain and 5 the worst imaginable pain.)
   0     1     2     3     4     5

8. *Where did you feel limited in your range of motion?*
   DAY 1:          _____
   DAY 15:         _____
   DAY 30:         _____

# AGING BACKWARDS FOR LIFE

Aging backwards is a way of life, not just a 30-day challenge. The Fast Track plan will set you on the path, knowing that you are the boss of your body and that it is designed to stay young if you choose to keep it that way. (Remember Way 6 and create a daily habit!)

Now that you've completed the 30-day program, what kinds of changes have you noticed in your body? Do you feel more relaxed, limber, less stiff? Do you have more energy? Do you feel stronger, better able to do work around the house? Do you find it easier to keep up with your colleagues or your (grand)kids? Have you been relieved of chronic pain? Record all of these changes in your diary, and compare them against when you started 30 days ago.

I hope that the Fast Track program has inspired you and given you the tools you need to enjoy a brighter future. Ideally it's a future even more exciting than the one you imagined before starting the plan—one in which you have all of the energy, strength, and confidence you need to tackle your goals (and dreams!) with confidence and vigor.

The rest of your life has only just begun—go out there and make the most of it! Are you prepared to commit to a life of aging backwards? I am, and I'm very glad I did!

Learn more about this program by visiting: www.essentrics.com/agingbackwards -fasttrack.

# ACKNOWLEDGMENTS

I n a book of this complexity, there are many people who have contributed above and beyond the call of duty to make this an innovative, interesting, and informative read. Although my name is on the cover, I consider all of the people listed equally deserving of credit for the part they have played in making this book happen; from writing, editing, photographing, and assembling. It was a massive undertaking.

It has been a pleasure working with this dedicated team, whom I am grateful to for their energy, enthusiasm, and grace in making this book a success. Each contributor deserves full acknowledgment for his or her participation in the making of this book.

I'd like to acknowledge and thank my dedicated agent, Ryan Harbage, who has been my greatest advocate in the publishing world. He is not just an agent but has played a guiding role in guaranteeing a quality manuscript was delivered to the publisher.

Finally, I wish to express my deep gratitude to Julie Will, my editor at Harper-Collins, and Anne Collins, my editor at Random House, for believing there is a place in this world for healthy aging and healthy exercising and for continuing to publish the *Aging Backwards* story. Thank you both for standing by me and supporting me as I try to shake up the world into understanding that aging doesn't have to be miserable and that serious exercising can be fun and easy.

EDITORS
Ryan Harbage
Julie Will, VP, Editorial Director, Harper Wave
Julia Pastore

WRITING AND RESEARCH ASSISTANTS
Lynn Moore
Gail Garceau
Amanda Cyr
Megan Feeney

PHOTOGRAPHY
Alexandre Paskanoi

DIRECTOR OF PHOTOGRAPHY
Elodie Nociti-Dubois

GRAPHIC DESIGN
Marwa Seif

CAPTIONING
Sasha Alcoloumbre
Francesca Esguerra
Tanya Escobar

INSTRUCTOR MODELS
Sahra Esmonde-White
Gail Garceau
Pierre-Luc Gagnon
Amanda Cyr
Megan Feeney

Thank you so much all of you.

*Miranda*

# NOTES

1. Helene Langevin, MD, CM, *Stretching, Connective Tissue, Inflammation, and Cancer*, Osher Center for Integrative Medicine video, 55:14, June 11, 2018, https://oshercenter.org/2018/06/11/video-stretching-connective-tissue-inflammation-and-cancer/.

2. Lisbeth Berrueta, Igla Muskaj, Sara Olenich, et al. "Stretching Impacts Inflammation Resolution in Connective Tissue," *Journal of Cellular Physiology*, 231, no. 7 (July 2016): 1621–27.

3. Petros C. Benias, Rebecca G. Wells, Bridget Sackey-Aboagye, et al. "Structure and Distribution of an Unrecognized Interstitium in Human Tissues," *Scientific Reports*, March 27, 2018, https://www.nature.com/articles/s41598-018-23062-6.pdf.

4. Helene M. Langevin, MD, CM, "The 'New Organ' in the News: Is It Real and What Does It Mean?" lecture, Osher Center for Integrative Medicine, Cambridge, MA, April 3, 2018. https://bwhedtech.media.partners.org/programs/integrative/integrative20180403langevin/.

5. Dean and Ayesha Sherzai, MD, *The Alzheimer's Solution: A Breakthrough Program to Prevent and Reverse the Symptoms of Cognitive Decline at Every Age* (San Francisco: HarperOne, 2017), p. 2.

6. J. A. Kleim, R. A. Swain, K. A. Armstrong, et al., "Selective Synaptic Plasticity Within the Cerebellar Cortex Following Complex Motor Skill Learning," *Neurobiology of Learning and Memory* 69, no. 3 (May 1998): 274–89.

7. A. Y. Klintsova, E. Dickson, R. Yoshida, and W. T. Greenough, "Altered Expression of BDNF and Its High-Affinity Receptor TrkB in Response to Complex Motor Learning and Moderate Exercise," *Brain Research* 1028, no. 1 (November 2004): 92–104.

8. "Pain Management," National Institutes of Health, last updated June 30, 2018. https://report.nih.gov/nihfactsheets/ViewFactSheet.aspx?csid=57.

9. http://www.painmed.org/patientcenter/facts_on_pain.aspx

10. M. Roig, K. O'Brien, G. Kirk, et al., "The Effects of Eccentric Versus Concentric Resistance Training on Muscle Strength and Mass in Healthy Adults: A Systematic Review with Meta-Analysis," *British Journal of Sports Medicine* 43, no. 8 (2009): 556–68.

11. Benjamin Gardner, Phillippa Lally, and Jane Wardle, "Making Health Habitual: The Psychology of 'Habit-Formation' and General Practice," *British Journal of General Practice* 62, no. 605 (December 2012): 664–66; https://www.ncbi.nlm.nih.gov/pmc/articles/PMC3505409/pdf/bjgp62–664.pdf.

12. Society for Personality and Social Psychology, "How We Form Habits, Change Existing Ones," ScienceDaily, www.sciencedaily.com/releases/2014/08/140808111931.htm (accessed September 25, 2018).

13. Leanna Skarnulis, "What's the Best Time to Exercise?," WebMD, https://www.webmd.com/fitness-exercise/features/whats-the-best-time-to-exercise#1.

14. "AAPM Facts and Figures on Pain," American Academy of Pain Medicine, http://www.painmed.org/patientcenter/facts_on_pain.aspx.

15. Melissa Conrad Stöppler, MD, "Hand Pain: Symptoms and Signs," Medicinenet, https://www.medicinenet.com/hand_pain/symptoms.htm.

16. M. J. Thomas, E. Roddy, W. Zhang, H. B. Menz, M. T. Hannan, and G. M. Peat, "The Population Prevalence of Foot and Ankle Pain in Middle and Old Age: A Systematic Review," *Pain* 152, no. 12 (December 2011): 2870–80.

17. A. Hruby and F. B. Hu, "The Epidemiology of Obesity: A Big Picture," *Pharmacoeconomics* 33, no. 7 (July 2015): 673–89.

18. Daniel J. Berry, MD, "First Nationwide Prevalence Study of Hip and Knee Arthroplasty Shows 7.2 Million Americans Living with Implants," Mayo Clinic, https://www.mayoclinic.org/medical-professionals/clinical-updates/orthopedic-surgery/study-hip-knee-arthroplasty-shows-7-2-million-americans-living-with-implants.

19. "Back Pain Facts and Statistics," American Chiropractic Association, https://www.acatoday.org/Patients/Health-Wellness-Information/Back-Pain-Facts-and-Statistics.

20. Leonardo Barbosa, Barreto de Brito, Djalma Rabelo Ricardo, et al, "Ability to Sit and Rise from the Floor as a Predictor of All-Cause Mortality," *European Journal of Preventive Cardiology*, 21 no. 7 (December 13, 2012): 892–98.

# INDEX

# ABOUT THE AUTHOR

MIRANDA ESMONDE-WHITE is the *New York Times* bestselling author of *Aging Backwards* and one of America's greatest advocates and educators of healthy aging. Following her career as a professional ballerina, Miranda developed her own fitness technique, Essentrics®, in 1997 and became the flexibility trainer to numerous professional and Olympic athletes and celebrities. Her top-rated fitness TV show, *Classical Stretch*, has been airing on PBS and Public Television since 1999, with the workouts available on DVD and streaming; and she offers fitness holidays and live teacher trainings at locations across the globe.

Esmonde-White's award-winning PBS documentaries, *Aging Backwards*, *Aging Backwards 2*, and *Forever Painless* are revolutionizing the way we understand the role that fitness plays in slowing down the aging process while keeping our bodies feeling young, strong, and healthy. She is also the author of *Forever Painless*, winner of a Nautilus Silver Book Award.